HEAR MY STRY
BEFORE I FORGET

HEAR MY STORY BEFORE I FORGET

THE TRAUMATIC JOURNEY OF A FORMER NFL PLAYER BATTLING A RARE BLOOD DISEASE AND EARLY-STAGE DEMENTIA WHO FINDS A RENEWED STRENGTH IN CHRIST

DARRYL CLACK

First Edition

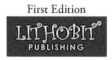

Hear My Story Before I Forget

Edited By: Lithobit Publishing

ISBN 978-0-578-49089-2
For speaking engagements, please visit www.darrylclack.com

Hear My Story Before I Forget
Published by Lithobit Publishing Copyright 2019
All rights reserved.

Contents

Preface

When a former NFL player, two-time high school Hall of Fame inductee, and the first freshman, in 1982, to lead the Arizona State University Sun Devils in rushing in 30 years, gets diagnosed with early-stage dementia and slips into a coma brought on by a life-threatening rare blood disease, life as he knew it changed forever.

"Hear My Story Before I Forget" chronicles Darryl Clack's celebrated sports journey, his coping mechanisms for multiple concussions, PTSD and depression, and journals the dark months of uncertainty that followed his traumatic illness and his fight to live.

A valuable tool for athletes, parents, sports fans or anyone suffering from an illness, that will aid in understanding how to detect symptoms of neurological damage, Thrombotic thrombocytopenic purport (TTP), concussions and other trauma related injuries. This book also discusses how young athletes in contact sports may protect themselves on the field and what measures to take to get help.

A narrative of inspiration, edification, and insight that unapologetically shows Darryl's renewed strength in Christ. Above all else, though, it is a memoir of faith, hope, healing, recovery, and transparency.

Thank you!

I want to give thanks first to God for keeping me safe and taking care of me and always being there no matter what issues or obstacles I face throughout my life.

I thank God for my successes and keeping me alive to experience my childhood dream of playing in the NFL with the Dallas Cowboys. I also thank Him for getting me through this journey with my illness. He is the reason for everything.

I want to thank my parents for everything they have done for me. Their love and prayers and all they sacrificed while allowing me to succeed in life.

Thank you to my brother, Cavanaugh, and sister, Vanessa for their support and prayers.

I thank my good friends and teammates for their unconditional support.

Thank you to my SportMetric family/business partners for having my back, updating my fans and friends on my progress and sharing my appreciation via social media.

I thank my wife Juanita and daughters Ashley and Darryana for their love, support, and patience during my illness, and being my number one fans. Thank you for dealing with my rollercoaster moments and being there through this journey.

Thank you to my publicist and publisher who has taken on this project and believed in me but most of all for being my friend, showing support, compassion, and understanding and for keeping me in God's word.

Thank you to the doctors and staff at Tri-City Medical on acting quickly and diagnosing me with TTP. Their knowledge, experience, and fight to keep me alive are much appreciated.

I also appreciate the hard work and determination of my doctors at the Mayo Clinic—Dr. John Camoriano, Dr. Jill Adamaski and her staff, and Dr. Nathan Delafield. They went beyond the call of duty to ensure my wellness. The Mayo Clinic staff is first class all the way.

Finally to football fans that still follow me and reach out to me, I appreciate all your support.

Warning-Disclaimer

This book is designed to edify and motivate and to provide information about TTP, concussions, dementia, sleep apnea, PTSD, depression. It is sold with the understanding that the publisher and author are not engaged in rendering legal or other professional services. If other expert assistance is required, the services of a competent professional should be sought.

You are urged to read all the available material, learn as much as you can about the above- mentioned illnesses, and tailor the information to your needs.

Through my experiences and research, every effort has been made to make this book as complete and as accurate as possible. However, there may be mistakes, both typographical and in content. Therefore, this book should be used only as a general guide and not as the ultimate source.

The purpose of this book is to complement, amplify and supplement other texts. The author and Lithobit Publishing shall have neither liability nor responsibility to any person or entity concerning any loss or damage caused, or allegedly caused, directly or indirectly, by the information contained in this book.

Introduction

Why me? What did I do to deserve this? What I thought would be a nice vacation with my family turned into a nightmare. One that I will never forget because October 10, 2016, is the day my entire life changed. It was the day I thought my life was over. The day that I realized I had no control over what would happen to me—whether I would live or die.

I awoke to a bright sunny morning and my family, and I hit the road to travel to San Diego for a vacation. The distance from Phoenix, Arizona to San Diego, CA is only six hours and 30 minutes (375 miles), so I knew we would be there in no time, and in enough time for me to get much-needed rest. After arriving in San Diego my family and I went for dinner and had a lovely time relaxing and preparing for the next day.

The next day the sun rose as usual, and I could smell the salt in the air from the ocean. It was a beautiful day, and I couldn't wait to hit the beach and to sink my feet into the sand— something I hadn't done in a while and was missing very much. We had a great time at the beach and later went to lunch. At lunch, we talked about going back to the beach and other plans for the next day.

I never had time to fulfill my plans the next day or even the next month because after lunch my life as I knew it changed forever. Proverbs 19:21 states, "You can make plans, but the Lord's purpose will prevail." Well, on that day, like every other day, the Lord's plan for me prevailed.

FIRST QUARTER: Growing Up Sports

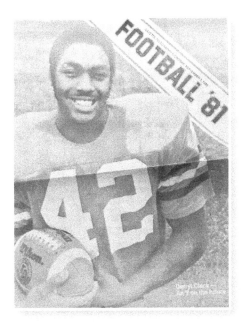

A llow me to introduce myself. My name is Darryl Clack, a young kid from San Antonio Texas, who loves the game of football. The start of my football career began in the second grade in a youth flag football program in Northern California.

My stay in California was short because as a military brat my dad was soon stationed in Kansas City, so naturally, my family and I moved to Kansas. I was in the fifth grade and that's when I started playing tackle football.

My positions were the quarterback and running back. One thing I did not realize about football was the amount of work and the constant hitting and tackling involved in the game. I did not like that so what did I do? I quit. My dad's rule was if you start something, you do your best and never give up. So he made me go back to finish what I started.

As time went on, I got used to the hard work required during practice and eventually started looking forward to game time. As the starting quarterback, throwing touchdown passes and running for touchdowns was a thrill, and the greatest feeling in the world was seeing and hearing all the people in the stands and on the sidelines, as well as my teammates and coaches screaming and cheering me on. I loved it.

All I wanted was to score touchdowns and win games, so I ran and ran as much as I could, and coaches kept giving me the ball, which seemed like every game.

One game I'll never forget is when I was running a sweep-right play—A running play where the quarterback takes the snap from center and then runs to the outside—and I took a head-on hit from the defender. I fell to the ground and lie there, and saw star-like fragments circling in my head, just like you see in cartoons.

My vision was blurred, and the coaches ran to check on me. They begin to ask me questions I could not answer because I could not remember anything. I started crying, and my parents came over to me on the sideline. Naturally, the coaches kept me out of the game.

My parents took me to the doctor, and after I was checked out, they drove me home, put me to bed and stayed by my side all night. Throughout the night my parents kept waking me up to check on me so that I would not slip into a coma or lose consciousness.

The next day my memory was back, and besides having a headache, I felt okay. So I went to practice the following week. This episode was my first experience of having a concussion, but it didn't deter me from playing the game I was growing to love.

Soon after, when I was in junior high school (middle school), my dad was stationed at Fort Carson, in Colorado Springs, CO. This meant that my family had to uproot once again. Because we moved there later in the school year, I missed the opportunity to be on the football team so, I started running track, I wrestled, played basketball, and I eventually joined the football team.

Although I played multiple sports in junior high school, the start of my success began in football and track. I played various positions in football, but I succeeded far more as a running back.

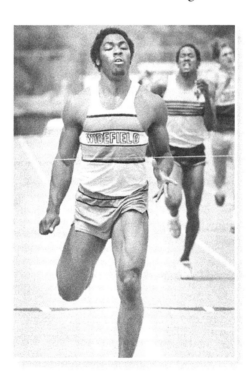

In track, I was winning —the 100-yard dash, 200-yard dash, long jump, triple jump, high jump, and 4x100 relay. I never lost a race. At the end of my junior high career, my dad received orders to transfer to Germany.

In my last year of junior high, at a track meet, a man approached me introducing himself as coach John Meese of Widefield High School. He told me I was a good athlete and asked me about my plans for high school. I wasn't sure but the two main high schools in the area were Fountain High and Widefield High.

The coach talked to my parents and told them about Widefield being state champions in track and top competitors in football and basketball.

My parents discussed my sports career in depth and realized I would have a better opportunity if I stayed in Colorado Springs. So, my mom, my younger brother and sister and I moved off the army base and to a suburb area called Security where I attended Widefield high school.

By the time I entered high school, my dad had been living in Germany for two years missing most of my high school football career. My "Supermom" was at all my football games along with working and raising my younger brother and sister.

On a spiritual side note, growing up I recall telling my mom that one day I would play in the NFL for the Dallas Cowboys and, I would buy her and my dad a new house and a new car because of the sacrifices they made for me to excel in sports—My way of saying thank you.

Mark 11:23 states, "...But you must believe it will happen and have no doubt in your heart. I tell you, you can pray for anything, and if you believe that you've received it, it will be yours."

I grew up in the church so knowing how to pray came naturally. I would pray every day and attend bible study weekly. I would ask God to guide my steps to make my dreams come true. I believed this would happen and I worked hard to achieve my goals.

My first year in high school was an excellent experience for my running track. We went to state and won the state championship in track. I won racing events, 200- yard dash, 400-yard dash 4x100 relay, 4x400 relay and had a photo finish in the 100-yard dash and took a close second. When I took second place, I was so upset that I made a promise to myself that I would never lose another race while in high school.

During football season my team went to the playoffs. We were very competitive in our division always winning games. In one game, as a running back, I took a handoff going off tackle and had a head-on collision with a linebacker causing me to have blurred vision and memory loss. I experienced my second concussion. By now I knew the routine-- out of the game, and to the hospital. The nurses took my vitals, and my parents monitored me throughout the night.

I continued to have a successful high school career such as winning three state championships in track, becoming high school athlete of the year, and All American in football and track. I kept my promise to myself, and I never lost a race in track during high school.

Concussion: What You Should Know

Experts refer to a concussion as a "mild traumatic brain injury," but it's not mild for anyone going through it, or to any parent taking care of a child who sustains one. A concussion can happen to anyone; however, most of the attention focuses on athletes, football in particular.

You previously read that I experienced concussions since the fifth grade from playing contact football. Just imagine not being able to remember anything that you know you should know and no matter how hard you try, you can't remember. It's a scary situation.

Here's a definition of concussion by Healthcare Leadership Blog:

Experts refer to a concussion as a "mild traumatic brain injury," but it's not mild for anyone going through it or to any parent taking care of a child who sustains one. A concussion can happen to anyone; however, most of the attention focuses on athletes, football in particular.

Typically, the brain (a very soft organ, similar to soft tofu) has adequate dual protection from the fluid that surrounds it (cerebrospinal fluid) and the boney skull that encases it. However, if our bodies or heads are subjected to a significant outside force, the brain shakes within and crashes into the skull. When this occurs, axons, the long slender projections of brain cells that carry messages, stretch and tear, producing characteristic symptoms, and leading to temporary functional impairment.

Through my company, SportMetric, the top objective is to make sure parents and players understand the protocol needed to be able to identify if a player or person may have a concussion.

Signs and Symptoms
of a Concussion

Children who are in organized sports have the luxury of having coaches, or even medical personnel on hand to make sure everything is okay after a blow to the head, but for those not in that situation, here are some signs and symptoms to look for:

- Physical symptoms
- Difficulty balancing
- Dizziness
- Headaches
- Increased fatigue
- Nausea
- Sensitivity to noise/light
- Trouble falling asleep
- Vision problems Cognitive symptoms
- Difficulty concentrating
- Difficulty remembering
- Feeling sluggish Emotional symptoms
- Extra emotional/moody
- Increased irritability
- Anxiety

What Every Youth Coach and Parent Should Know and Do

The Centers for Disease Control and Prevention (CDC) lists six action steps that parents and youth coaches should take if they think a child sustains a concussion:

1. Learn how to recognize a concussion. To identify a concussion, you should look for two things:
    a) A blow to the head or to the body that moves the head violently
    b) Any sign or symptom that indicates a change in the child's physical, cognitive, emotional function or behavior.

2. Learn the Danger Signs of brain injury:
    *   One pupil is more significant than the other.
    *   Drowsiness or inability to wake up.
    *   A headache that gets worse and does not go away.
    *   Slurred speech, weakness, numbness, or decreased coordination.

- Repeated vomiting or nausea, convulsions or seizures (shaking or twitching).
- Unusual behavior, increased confusion, restlessness, or agitation.
- Loss of consciousness (passed out/knocked out). Even a brief loss of consciousness must be addressed seriously.

3. Remove the child from play and obtain a medical evaluation. Do not try to judge the seriousness of the injury yourself.

4. Support proper treatment. After a concussion, the individual's brain should not be over-stimulated. The less "work" the brain has to do, especially early in recovery, the more energy it can put toward healing. It is essential to provide a careful balance between activity and rest, not allowing the symptoms to worsen.

5. Use tools to guide your recognition and response. The CDC materials are excellent, either in paper form or via the Concussion Recognition & Response (CRR) app to help guide your recognition of the signs and symptoms (Children's National).

The Home Symptom Monitoring feature of the CRR app can assist you to track symptom progress and provide this valuable information to support post-injury treatment.

Parents, you have every right to be worried anytime your child gets on the field to play any sports, in particular, football. For peace of mind and to ensure that safety is the priority of the sports organization, do your due diligence by asking specific questions.

RiseandShine.com suggests the following 10 questions:

1. Does the league have a general policy on how they manage concussions?
2. Does the league have access to healthcare professionals with knowledge and training in sport- related concussion?
3. Are the coaches required to take a concussion education and training course?
4. Who is responsible for the sideline concussion recognition and response to suspected concussions during practice and games?
5. Do the coaches have readily available the tools — concussion signs & symptoms cards, clipboards, fact sheets, and smart-phone apps during practice and games to guide proper recognition and response of a suspected concussion?
6. Does the league provide concussion education for the parents, and what is the policy for informing parents of suspected concussions?
7. What is the policy regarding allowing a player to return to play? [Correct answer – when an appropriate medical professional provides written clearance that the athlete is fully recovered and ready to return.]
8. Does the league teach/coach proper techniques (e.g., blocking and tackling in football, checking in hockey and lacrosse) in a way that is "head safe" by not putting the head in position to be struck? If the player does demonstrate unsafe technique during practice or a game, do the coaches re-instruct them with the proper procedure/method? Are head and neck strengthening taught?
9. If a contact sport, are there limitations to the amount of contact? How often (# days per week, # minutes per practice) do you practice with live contact? Is that any different than past years?

10. How amenable is the league/team/coach to accepting feed-back from parents about their child's safety as it relates to head protection?

I'd never heard of the Right Eye Test until I read an article on Techcrunc.com by Devin Coldewey entitled, "Righteye's Portable Eye-Tracking Test Catches Concussions and Reading Problems in Five Minutes." Right-eye is a portable device that tests for effects of concus-sions or other traumas on the playing field and gives players a chance to get immediate help by testing early.

Coldewey states, "A basic EyeQ (as they call it) test takes five min-utes or so, with more specialized tests adding only a few more, and results are available immediately." This test could be the difference in saving a life because, after one concussion or hit, players are susceptible to more damage to the brain if allowed to return to the field.

Another article that I feel is important to mention is on Webmd.com entitled, "One-Minute Sideline Test Predicts Concussions." It ex-plains how a simple eye test can detect a concussion.

The test is simple. Before the game, a coach or trainer shows an athlete a set of three index cards. Each card has a series of numbers scattered across eight lines. The athlete reads the numbers from left to right. After a blow to the head, the athlete goes to the sidelines and retakes the test. If he's five seconds slower, he may have suffered a concussion—and is at serious risk if his head gets hit again. The test is performed because it turns out that eye movement links to neurological function. Who knew?

When is it safe to return to the field?

Any student who shows signs, symptoms, and behaviors consistent with a concussion should be immediately removed from any activity and be evaluated by the team or school medical provider, if available, and if not, by the coach or other designated person.

No student should return to physical activity on the same day if a concussion is suspected. Nor should a student return to action after an apparent head injury or concussion, regardless of how mild it seems or how quickly symptoms clear, without written medical clearance from a health care provider.

According to TN Senate Bill 882, if an athlete suffers, or is suspected of having experienced, a concussion or head injury during a competition or practice, the athlete must be immediately removed from the competition or practice and cannot return to play or participate in any supervised team activities involving physical exertion, including games, competitions or practices, until an approved health care provider evaluates the youth athlete and receives written clearance from the authorized health care provider for a full or graduated return to play.

As a parent or student, you must take heed of this information. Although I'm not saying it will prevent concussions from happening, however, it could be what you need to get help faster in the event a concussion does occur. However, remember the golden rule, when in doubt, sit them out!

Arizona State University

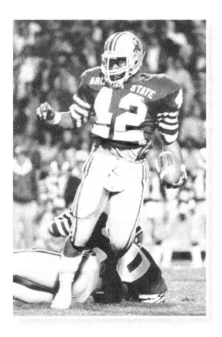

My concussions did not deter me from playing football. I loved the game and expected to get a full scholarship to a four-year university where I would continue playing. As I completed my final year in high school, I had opportunities to attend many universities throughout the country, such as Notre Dame, SMU, Arkansas, University of Colorado, University of Arizona, University of Oklahoma, UCLA, USC, LSU, University of Texas, Arizona State University, Stanford, and many more.

My first choice was Notre Dame. So obviously, I had to visit the school to see if it was the right fit. On the day of my visit, I was in the Denver airport waiting for a flight to South Bend Indiana, but they had a snowstorm and delayed all flights. At that point, I decided to forego my trip. Not to reschedule, but to take Notre Dame out of the running altogether.

It was at that moment that I knew I had no interest in living in another state where it snowed because when I thought about it, being in Colorado since junior high school and dealing with the snow, wasn't so appealing. I needed to be at a school where the climate was warm.

I also needed to be at a university that would not only give me a chance to play as a freshman but also allow me to run track so, I chose Arizona State University (ASU). ASU had a gorgeous campus, excellent facilities, great weather and a football team with a winning track record.

The cherry on top was that I would be able to run track as well. So I accepted a football scholarship to attend Arizona State University and began to play as a freshman running back with much success.

I now understand the meaning of Proverbs 16:9 explicitly, "We can make our plans, but the Lord determines our steps." I was so ready to attend Notre Dame, but God had other plans. His plan was for me to attend ASU.

Once at ASU, most of my freshman class I redshirted so I thought I would redshirt for the remaining season, but that was not the case. I recall our game against the Oregon Ducks. During the game Coach, Darryl Rogers called me over to replace Tex Wright, the starting fullback. Now here is the catch.

At the time my position was a tailback, and I'd never played fullback in my life, meaning, I'm not a blocker nor do I know the fullback plays. So I must admit I was scared as heck when the opportunity presented itself.

Now, I knew the coaches knew this wasn't my position, and I

contemplated reminding them of my lack of experience as a fullback, but it was in the heat of the moment, so I kept my mouth shut and went in the game. To my surprise, the coach called six straight running plays to me, and I ran like my life depended on it.

When the game was over, I learned that I had led the team in rushing which led to the start of my career at Arizona State. When I completed the season, I was the first freshman in 30 years to lead the team in rushing and was on the verge of having a promising collegiate career.

In another game, we were playing UCLA, and I took a handoff up the middle and took a hit on the back of my head. I remember getting up and walking to the huddle; my quarterback called the next play. I had no clue as to what I was doing so I asked the quarterback, "What do I do?" He told me what to do.

After, I went back to the huddle, and the quarterback called another play. Once again, I did not remember what to do so I asked him again, "What do I do?" Once again he told me the play, but this time he called a timeout and went to the sideline to express his concerns to the coaches because he thought something was wrong.

The coaches brought me over to the sideline and began to check my eyes. They asked me many questions that I could not remember. One, in particular, was, "Do you know where you are?" I answered, "No." Another question was, "What are your parent's names?" I could not remember. That scared me enough to stay out of the game even if the coaches hadn't demanded.

What's strange is that I thought nothing was wrong with me while I was playing because I was doing a great job on the field and making all the plays. However, after thinking about it days later, I realized that I was making the plays off instinct.

I played the following week and continued to play throughout my college career. I sustained numerous injuries such as hip pointers, turf toe, bruised ribs, ankle injuries, knee injuries, and stingers to name a few. I continued to lead the team in rushing, and in my freshman year, we played at the University of Oklahoma in the Fiesta Bowl and won the game.

In my second year, I lead the team in rushing. We had a good year and was selected as second team all PAC 10 conference.

In my third year, another good year, I led the team in rushing and led the conference in yards per game and was selected to the all PAC 10 conference. I was selected as Arizona State University's offensive player of the year and as MVP.

In my fourth year, a new coach joined the staff. Coach John Cooper took the place of my former coach, Darryl Rogers who accepted a coaching position with the Detroit Lions.

I only needed 1500 yards to be Arizona State University's all-time leading rusher. However, during the third game of the season, I took a hit and landed on my leg wrong which caused me to miss the rest of the game.

It seemed to be a high ankle sprain but, as time went on and many days of treatment, it was not healing. I kept telling the trainers and coaches that there was something wrong with my leg. I had X-rays done, but they did not reveal anything. I kept trying to play but my leg was not getting any better, so I continued to stress that something was seriously wrong with my leg.

The impression the coaches had put out there was that I wouldn't play injured. In football, the motto is, "If you can't play with pain, you can't play the game," but that was not the case. Nothing could be further from the truth. I played injured many times even times when no one knew I was hurt, but I could tell something was not right with my leg.

At that point, I felt that the coaching staff and trainers were not looking out for me, so I had to look out for myself. I'm a college athlete in a state with no family, and since my coaches weren't taking my injury serious, I called my mom who worked in the medical field.

She flew in from Texas and took me to Tempe Hospital. The doctor ordered an MRI scan for my leg that revealed I had a stress fracture in my right fibula. My leg was placed in a cast and sadly my football season was over.

I did not get any apologies from the coaching staff, trainers or medical staff at ASU. I was a bit upset with them for not looking at other options to determine why my injury was not healing.

At that point, I had mixed emotions towards them all, and mixed feelings about taking a medical hardship to stay at ASU another year—a fifth year.

For those of you who do not understand how the option works to stay at a four-year university and play five years, I'll explain.

When a school brings in a college athlete on a full-ride scholarship, the NCAA rule is that the athlete has five years to get in four full years of playtime.

First, if that player is put on a redshirt year their first year, they will not play in a regular game at all during that year. Meaning the team does not need the player at that specific time because they have enough coverage for that particular position or they feel that the player has room for improvement, saving the player for the next year. The player will be there for five years but will play only four full years.

Since I did not redshirt the first year and played as a freshman, it meant that I would be there and play four years, but because my injury was in my fourth year, I could not play a full fourth year.

The other option would be for me to go on medical hardship, which meant due to medical reasons I could not play my fourth and final year. Remember, each player gets five years to play four years so if I took a medical hardship that meant I would get another year to play once I was well. However, I decided to bypass the medical hardship and go into the NFL draft.

I have no regrets about my college years. Yeah, I worked hard on the field, but I had a great time off the field as well. I had great friends, some of whom I still keep in touch, and my experiences and memories are priceless.

My college life was such a fun and exciting time in my life, and it made me wiser and smarter on and off the field.

As I stated, I had real friends, but I also had "new friends" who only wanted to be around when I was flying high.

I was blessed to be on a billboard ad. At that time, Arizona did not have a professional football team, so the Sun Devils were it. We were the football stars of the state. So me being on a billboard for all to see was a big deal.

I also used to give awesome parties where at least 200 people would show up and pay to get in. Looking back, I knew why I had new "friends," but I learned that it came with the territory and more importantly I knew how to handle them accordingly.

My time in college also helped me become more disciplined in life. Here's an example of my college schedule. Keep in mind that I was a two-sport athlete at Arizona State University.

During the football season, I would start my day going to all my classes starting at 7:00 am. The rule is we had to have a minimum of 12 hours per semester, which are about four classes.

After my classes, I would go to the athletic department to get ready for football meetings for about 2-3 hours. After, I had to get dressed and taped up for football practice that lasted from around 3:00 pm until about 5:30 pm.

Then, I would go back to get treatment, shower, dress, and on some occasions would have another quick football meeting to look at practice films.

After films, we had dinner around 6:00 pm, and after I would have study hall with tutors until around 8:00 or 9:00 pm. At that point, my day was over.

However, my day could go longer depending on my class and study major for example I was a computer science major. I had lab assignments and would have to go to the computer lab, register to get a computer and wait until one was available to complete homework. So, in reality, I would get done by 11:00 p.m. Because of the grueling schedule and a few other reasons, I ended up changing my major. Ridiculous!

NCAA rules require each athlete to maintain a 2.0 GPA. At any point, if a player falls below that GPA, it could cost them not to play and lose their football scholarship. With all the things football players were required to do, it was exhausting. But I looked at it this way; I'm getting a free education and playing a game I love. Why not take advantage of the benefits and focus on getting a college degree?

Although my schedule was full, I still had time to enjoy my college life—parties, friends, and a few relationships. It's about balance and getting an education because there is life after the game. The term to never forget is student-athlete, meaning student first, and then athlete second.

Dallas Cowboys
Here I Come!

At the end of my collegiate career, I was drafted by the Dallas Cowboys as a running back and kick returner in the second pick of the second round.

As I previously stated, when I was in high school I told my parents I wanted to play in the NFL and play for the Dallas Cowboys, buy them a new house and a new car. Ladies and Gentlemen, I'm an example of how dreams come true through the will of God. He granted my prayers. I played in the NFL for the Dallas Cowboys, and I bought my parents a brand new house and a new

Mercedes. When the Cowboys drafted me, the understanding was that I would be a backup for the famous Hall of Famer, and my idol, Tony Dorsett, but there was a setback. Herschel Walker decided to leave the USFL. The Dallas Cowboys owned his rights, so he came back to play with the Cowboys.

That put me further back on the depth chart—a list of players per position that will show how many players you have for that position. For example, when the Cowboys drafted me they had Tony Dorsett as number one, and I would be number two, and another player would be number three and so on.

When Herschel Walker joined the team, I dropped to number three on the chart, and he became number two. Each football team will only keep a certain amount of players per position and usually for the running back position they may retain a total of four players. My bubble soon deflated.

Now I'm behind two Heisman trophy winners and Hall of Famers; however, it was an honor to be on the team and to be on the same field as players I grew up watching. Tony Dorsett, Tony Hill, Too Tall Jones, Randy White, Danny White, and Everson Walls are a few of many, and being part of the Cowboy family with Roger Stabauch, Drew Pearson, Bob "The Bullet" Hayes, Ron Springs, and Robert Newhouse was priceless. What are the odds?

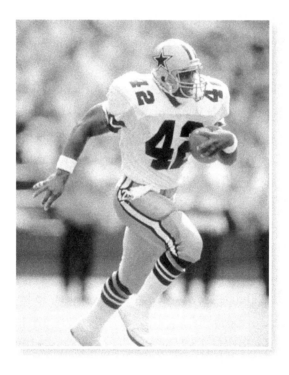

My career with the Dallas Cowboys was mainly as a kickoff returner and special teams, and at times I backed up Tony Dorsett or Herschel Walker.

I remember my first game was in London against the 1985 super bowl champs Chicago Bears. We marched down the field, and we were on the goal line. I took a handoff from Danny White off tackle and while heading into the end zone out of nowhere Mike Singletary, all-pro linebacker, got free and hit me on my left shoulder.

I fumbled the ball and left the game with a separated shoulder. I said to myself, "that's just great." My first year, and first game and now I may be out for the year. I decided there is no way I'm going to be out my first year, so I continued to play the remainder of the year with an injured shoulder.

Throughout the year, every so often, I would take a good hit on my shoulder, and it would pop out, and I would have to get it put back in place. I must admit the pain was very excruciating. At the end of the year, I had surgery to repair my shoulder, and I would continue to play my second and third year.

In my third year, the San Diego Chargers contacted the Cowboys about a trade for me to go to San Diego which I was all for but, the Cowboys said they had plans for me and would not make the deal. Exciting, right? I thought so, but another setback happened.

Jerry Jones purchased the Cowboys, and Jimmy Johnson from the University of Miami became the new head coach. No more Tom Landry. My plans with the Dallas Cowboys went out the door with Landry.

The franchise made numerous trades such as Herschel Walker going to the Minnesota Vikings and decided to release me without renewing my contract.

Getting released was a horrible feeling to experience. I worked hard all year. I trained hard, attended all mini-camps then moved on to regular camp. I played in all pre-season football games. I played in over half of the regular season games, then all of a sudden, I get asked to see the head coach, Jimmy Johnson. He stated that due to the changes they were making within the team, they felt I would not be a good fit, so they released me allowing me to shop around for other teams.

It was a sad feeling that went through my entire body, and a lump in the pit of my stomach weighed heavy. I began to question my ability and work ethic. I had hoped to play my entire career with the Dallas Cowboys, but I realized this was the nature of the business.

Football players are useful in their prime. As they get older, their talents start to diminish. Injuries begin to occur, and before we know it, a younger player comes in healthier and stronger and, it's time for us to look for another job.

My agent, Bruce Allen, shopped me around to other teams. I had tryouts with Buddy Ryan and the Philadelphia Eagles, and with Don Shula and the Miami Dolphins, but I ended up signing a new contract with the Cleveland Browns because they made a better contract offer. As I mentioned earlier, this is a business, and we go to the best offer.

Once in Cleveland, I reported to all minicamps, and when preseason started, I had a pretty good camp experience. Then I was injured and had to miss a pre-season game. Well, once again this is a business, and when you are hurt and can't play, it's not a good situation. I made it until the final cut and was released. I started to second-guess my abilities once more.

Reoccurring injuries were starting to take its toll and happening too often, so I decided it was time to end my career.

As fate would have it, I got a call from the General Manager of the Toronto Argonauts, from the Canadian Football league, offering me a one-year contract. I decided to give it one more shot and accepted the offer.

I packed my bags and caught a flight to Toronto. The move was the right decision because the team was outstanding and we won the 1991 Grey Cup championship defeating the Calgary Stampeders 36-21. The Grey Cup is similar to the Super Bowl of the NFL.

For those of you who are not familiar with the Canadian football league, each city in Canada has a team of American and Canadian football players and coaches. Wayne Gretzky and John Candy were part owners of the Toronto Argonauts.

This league had been around longer than the NFL, so I was able to get a championship ring after all. What a great feeling and a way to top off my football career! Toronto is such a great city, and I had a great time living there.

After my contract was up, I returned home, and before I could settle in I received a call from coach Pete Levine to play for head coach Galen Hall for one season in the NFL World League—a league established by the NFL. In the World League, each team is made up of NFL players from different NFL teams. We played games throughout the states and Europe. I played for the Orlando Thunder located in Orlando Florida.

What I liked about this league was that it brought the fun back into football. There were no contract negotiations to deal with because each contract was a set amount based on the position. It was great because not only was I having a great time playing the game that I love, with a great team, I was traveling on an all-expense-paid tour through Europe, courtesy of the NFL.

I had a great year leading my team in rushing and touchdowns. I was also top in the league in rushing and touchdowns and voted "All World." The Orlando Thunder was a good team so it wasn't surprising that we would play for the 1992 World Bowl championship against the San Antonio team where we were runner-up.

I played great; however, my injuries had gotten worse during the season. They were so unbearable that I was taking pain pills before and after practice to be able to tolerate the discomfort.

In the meantime, some NFL teams were looking at me to return to the NFL, but I realized there was no way I could keep dealing with all the pain in both of my knees and ankles, and the injury of cracked ribs.

Between all the injuries and head trauma from playing with the

Dallas Cowboys, Cleveland Browns, Toronto Argonauts, and Orlando Thunder, in addition to doctors telling me I would have to have surgery on my knees if I wanted to continue to play, I decided to retire for good. I'd had enough. Besides, according to doctors, at the rate I was going, there was a good chance I would have to depend on a walker to get around, in my later years.

SECOND QUARTER: Get It Together, Clack!

After my playing days in football, not knowing what I wanted to do and not having a plan B, I was lost. I was financially unstable. Granted I did not make money like football players today, but it was good money, and it would have lasted; however, I lost a lot of money on a bad investment.

So what do most people do when they need to reboot their lives? If they're blessed enough to have loving and caring parents, who are still living, they move home. Yep. You got it. I moved back to El Paso, Texas where my parents were living—they were stationed at Fort Bliss Army Base and had decided to make it home after I graduated from high school.

Moving in with my parents was a blessing, and it was a safe place for me to figure out my next move, but instead of being motivated and mapping out my plan, I became depressed about my football career not turning out how I had hoped.

I started gambling. I was searching for that rush I felt while playing football. I was not hearing the screams and people calling my name anymore from the stands in the stadium. I was not getting the attention I received while playing the game. Football was all I knew. Football was my life. I had a reason to wake up. For years I had a purpose and a daily blueprint to follow.

My life was very structured when I played football. For example, I would train four to five hours a day seven days a week, preparing for the season. From April to June mini camps were one to two weeks where plays were practiced to prepare for the July/August camp.

During camp our wake up time was 6:00 am. I would have breakfast, attend a meeting at 7:00 am, and from there I would get ready to be on the field for the first practice at 9:00 am that lasted for 2 to 2.5 hours.

After the first practice, I would get any treatment needed, then go to lunch at 1:00 pm. After, I would take a break and maybe get a nap in before the start of second practice that started at 3:00 pm. for another 2 to 2.5 hours.

After practice, once again, I had more treatment, if needed, then dinner at 6:00 pm and off to a meeting at 7:00 pm to go over practice footage. My day would end by 8:30 p.m. and I would have free time until 11:00 p.m. curfew. This process would repeat five days straight to include a preseason game, following one day off. This schedule would last for four weeks until the season began.

Let's talk about the start of the season. Games on Sunday, depending on the time of the game, I would wake up, have breakfast, have a meeting, then off to the stadium I'd go to get ready for the game. After the game and all press interviews, the team would go to the airport, if it wasn't a home game, and fly back home.

Because of the traveling and the long day on Sunday, on Monday I wouldn't have to check in until 8:00 am for treatments, workout, and then meetings to go over the game film and to discuss the upcoming week. Usually, my day was over by noon.

Tuesday was my day off and Wednesday I'd start the process all over again until the end of the season. I dedicated every day to stay at the top of my game.

This schedule is an example of how defined my life was throughout my entire football career. I loved football, and I had no other interest.

So when I retired—the transition to retirement had its challenges—I didn't have that one thing I loved anymore nor did I have a daily plan: no structure in my life and no noise from the crowds in the stadium. No purpose. It was too quiet. The only question that continuously popped into my head was, "Now what?"

The more I tried to figure out where I would get back that type of life, the deeper it took me into depression. I had mood swings and became very angry and unhappy. I shut down and started questioning God about what was happening. I couldn't understand how I could go from being so happy and fulfilling most of my dreams, to having to start my life over.

Depression

Depression is a common and serious health problem that affects millions of people. It's an illness that affects people's thoughts, feelings, emotions, and believe it or not, physical health. According to "The Trust," about 12% of all men are expected to have at least one significant episode of depression in their lifetime, and there is growing evidence that former professional football players may be at increased risk for depression.

After football, I experienced and still experience depression and factors associated with depression such as sleep apnea, chronic pain, anxiety, social withdrawal, mood swings, irritability, and memory loss.

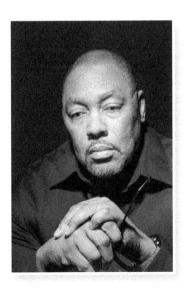

Several studies have looked at the connection between concussions and depression in high-performance athletes in contact sports. According to the article "How Connected Are Concussions and Depression?" the main findings are that those that suffer from multiple concussions have a higher risk of depression.

In dealing with depression, doctors want to prescribe antidepressants immediately. If I can help it, I will not add another pill to my daily regimen. I've opted to counter some of my symptoms without prescription meds. Here are a few alternatives:

- Cut Back on Caffeine – stimulants keep you awake
- Get More Sleep – getting the right amount of sleep at the same time each night
- Get More Vitamin D - getting enough sunshine is key
- Spirituality – coming closer to God and reminding myself how grateful I am daily
- Exercise – daily low-intensity exercise to include outdoor activity
- Cut Out Alcohol – alcohol is a depressant
- Diet – eating a well-balanced diet is key
- Stay Social – it's good to make plans with friends and family to laugh, socialize and stay active
- Yoga – improves mood and relaxation

I have yet to try acupuncture and support groups but I haven't ruled them out.

The Fumble

In football, a fumble occurs when a player who has possession and control of the ball loses it before being tackled or scoring. Looking back, I realize that everything that was going downhill for me—depression, injuries, bad investments, and being cut from the Cowboys and the Browns--were because my focus on and relationship with God was lacking.

When things are going well, we forget to continue our relationship with God. Often we forget that the devil is looking for opportunities to harm us and take us away from God. He is watching our every move and waiting for opportunities to strike. It is imperative that even in the good times, we still have a relationship with God.

In my case, I was not spending my time daily in God's word. If I could study the football playbook daily, I certainly could have picked up a bible and spent quality time with God.

James 5:13 states, "Are any of you suffering hardships? You should pray. Are any of you happy? You should sing praise." In bad times it's automatic that we pray, but we should also pray in good times. In fact, we should worship God and give Him thanks 24/7.

The Bible displays many examples of how the devil will try to tempt us. In Matthew 3:16-17 John baptizes Jesus. Shortly after, in Matthew 4:1, the devil tempted Jesus to try to lead him off course. This example tells us that in times when we're feeling safe and secure, we need to be on our toes even more because as the saying goes, "The devil is busy." Busy trying to tempt anyone who loses focus on God—waiting to lead us astray.

Fumble Recovery

Fumble recovery is when an offensive player in possession of the ball fumbles and either team recovers the ball. Fumble recovery is counted even when the same team that fumbled regains possession.

2 Timothy 2 (NLT) is entitled "A good soldier for Christ Jesus." In 2 Timothy 2:5 the bible states, "…Athletes cannot win the prize unless they follow the rules." I wasn't following the rules. I wasn't in God's word daily nor was I living a Christ-like life. In my mind, I had it all—cars, houses, money, and I was on one of the best teams in the NFL. I was living my dream and enjoying my blessings.

My fumble recovery was when I decided to regain possession of my life. I needed to figure out why things were not going well for me and to try to make it right. This time, I needed God to guide my journey.

My Purpose Driven Journey

To my understanding, when you do something with purpose, you do it with determination. As a football player, I was determined, focused and followed my passion; therefore, I fulfilled my purpose. After football, I had to figure out how to live a passion-filled life on purpose.

One day my mom reached out to me because she was concerned about my wellbeing. She strongly suggested that I get back in church and reminded me that the only reason I had any success was that of God. I took her advice and started going back to church and made a decision to be re-baptized.

I felt I needed to do this because my first baptism was when I was seven years old and although we were in church and Sunday school every Sunday, at that age, I didn't quite understand the meaning behind baptism.

Since I was starting my life over and was asking God for forgiveness to help me get my life back on track, getting baptized again with a better understanding seemed right.

My prayer was also for God to take away the depression that was so deeply rooted in me and to help me find purpose in my life. The Bible tells us to be filled with joy and praise (Philippians 4:4; Romans 15:11). God intends for us all to live joyful lives. I knew this would not be an easy fete, but through prayer, bible study and application, confession, and forgiveness my prayers were answered.

We never know how fast our prayers are met or what the blessing will be to complement our prayer. God has a funny way of getting us on track when we least expect it. During my time of prayer and asking God to get me out of my funk, the Colorado Sports Hall of Fame announced my 1993 induction.

This induction was the start of my comeback. Being inducted gave me back my mojo. I was once again on a platform where people applauded me and acknowledged my accomplishments. Just, the jolt I needed.

God started to reveal many things to me in particular, why I should be thankful. He also made me realize my purpose in life—to rediscover myself, fulfill my happiness, make a positive difference, evolve spiritually, and to cultivate my God-given gifts. I make it sound like it was easy to reinvent myself, regain my confidence, and face the world as a former NFL player, but it wasn't.

It took a while but I finally snapped out of it and boy it felt good. I was back. I had my swag, my confidence and nothing was going to stop me from fulfilling my new purposes. Yep! I had several reasons to live and several dreams to fulfill. D.C. was back! I had a renewed mind, and a desire to want to get out of bed to be productive. What a blessing.

I remember promising my parents that no matter what, I would get my college degree. So I registered at the University of Texas at El Paso (UTEP) and worked on completing my undergraduate degree.

During that time I also decided to look for a job. I did not have any work experience because my only job was to play football. I applied for a sales manager position with Nordic Track, and they hired me! Looking back, I shouldn't have been surprised. I was a former professional football player, and if anyone knew sports, exercise equipment, and overall body conditioning, it was I.

However, because I was slowly starting to get my confidence back, I was positively surprised but grateful. It was my first ever job interview and my first management position. I was in charge of managing a team in selling exercise equipment. How appropriate.

The company sent me to their corporate office in Minnesota for training, and when I returned to El Paso, I was up and running. As I look back, I can't believe how ordinary my life became. I was now a regular student in school (not a jock) and working a regular job. No more football or track practice, and all the benefits that came with being a professional athlete disappeared. This new life felt weird, and it took some time to adjust.

Two years later after working very hard in school and at Nordic Track, I received a Bachelor of Science degree in Kinesiology and Sports Studies. I was so excited about my accomplishment! It boosted my confidence and motivated me so much that I continued my education and without a break, I enrolled in the University of Phoenix and started working towards a Masters of Arts degree in Organizational Management.

I then applied for a job as an assistant store manager at Champs Sports and was hired. This time I wasn't surprised. I nailed the interview, and I also had experience under my belt. I continued getting management experience while going to school full time.

During my journey, I met a guy who worked for a residential treatment center for teens. These facilities offer a range of services, including drug and alcohol treatment, confidence building, discipline, and psychological counseling for a variety of addiction, emotional, and behavioral problems. Many of the programs are intended to provide a less constricting option to imprisonment or hospitalization.

The guy explained to me how he mentored teens and how his job was very fulfilling. I thought it would be something worth researching.

Remember, all I knew was football and even though I had two jobs after football, and excelled in my management positions, at this point in my life I was still finding my way through and seeking a purpose for my future. I had my manager position at Champs; however, I wanted to help kids and give back because that is what I'd always done through the NFL.

I applied for the position at the residential treatment center, and they hired me as a counselor. It was a great, humbling experience working with the kids and helping them figure out their problems. The most significant and most rewarding experience for me was witnessing kids whom I worked with finally leave the treatment center, and go on to be law-abiding citizens.

They would reach out to thank me for helping them get over their hurdles and update me on their success—graduating from high school, attending college or working a fulltime job. Those phone calls would make my day. Knowing that I had a hand in helping troubled kids overcome their issues and excel in life was the best feeling ever. Moreover, I fulfilled one of my purposes along the way.

Now if you recall, I was working fulltime at Champs Sports as a manager, part-time at the residential treatment center and was a fulltime student. My hands were full, but I stayed focused. Two years later, I graduated with a Master's degree in Organizational Management—another accomplishment under my belt.

Feeling good about myself, extremely motivated and ready to take my education and job experience to the next level, I applied for a position at Brylane Inc., a catalog company for different retail organizations such as Sears, Lane Bryant, Chadwicks of Boston, Brylane Home, and King Size Big and Tall.

They were preparing to open locations in Texas. They hired me as a supervisor to oversee a team of 100 representatives and two Team Leaders in their King Size Big and Tall department. I was very successful in this position. I met all my sales goals and had a great rapport with everyone.

After such a good year, I was promoted to call center business manager in charge of running the largest department in the company called Chadwicks of Boston. I managed a total of 400 representatives, four team-leaders, and two supervisors. I had a great team, and I was ready and well prepared to move up even higher within the company.

On a beautiful September day in 2001, I was scheduled to travel to New York for a company meeting where I had a layover flight in Houston, Texas. After boarding the plane and finding my seat preparing to endure the last leg of the trip, the aircraft pushed back and taxied on the ground at a low speed. I noticed that it was taking a very long time for the plane to hit the runway and take off. What seemed like an hour later, possibly due to my anticipation of arriving in New York, was only 20 minutes when the captain announced that the flight was being rerouted back to the gate, with no explanation.

Arriving back to the gate, still with no explanation, we sat there a while longer when the Captain finally announced that everyone had to abort the plane and that no aircraft would be flying to New York for the remaining day.

As I deplaned and entered the airport, I noticed people frantically looking at the TV monitors while on their phones. When I looked up to see what was going on, I was in shock. I will never forget what I saw on the monitor. It was something out of a movie because airplanes were crashing into buildings in New York. The United States was under attack. It was 9/11!

I was in an airport in Houston, TX away from family and friends. All flights canceled and all airports closed. As I watched these haunting attacks, I remember sitting in the airport crying in disbelief and shocked that something like this was happening. I was so upset not knowing what to do or how to help. I felt useless. One thing for sure, I was stranded along with thousands of other scared people not knowing what would happen next.

After spending a couple of days in Houston, the airport reopened, and I was finally able to catch a flight back to El Paso. Arriving back to the same airport, three days after the September 11th terrorist attacks, was eerie. Walking through the terminal was uneasy and morbid. The happy faces greeting loved ones and people laughing and talking three days ago was no more. This time people were subdued and unsure. I was undoubtedly uneasy and anxious to get back home.

When I boarded my flight, the atmosphere understandably was depressing. A one-hour and 50- minute trip from Houston, Texas to El Paso, Texas felt like five hours. It was torcher. However, I was alive. I was going home to see my loved ones, but I kept thinking about all the victims killed, and I couldn't help but feel sad.

When the plane landed in El Paso, it was such a good feeling to be back home, and I was so thankful to be alive. In Psalm 138:7 (NLT) the bible says, "Though I am surrounded by troubles, you will protect me from the anger of my enemies. You reach out your hand, and the power of your right hand saves me."

If you weren't paying attention earlier, I mentioned that my flight to New York was on September 11, 2001. I was scheduled to land in New York City the same day terrorists attacked the city. The deadliest terrorist attack on U.S. soil in U.S. history! God spared my life.

Going Back to A.Z.

After spending five years with Brylane, Inc., I decided to move back to Phoenix, Arizona. Even though my career was taking off and I earned two degrees, there was still something missing. I always felt the need to be back in Phoenix. It was my stomping ground where I had great memories of football and friends. It's sort of like the sitcom "Cheers" where everybody knows your name.

So I took a leap of faith, submitted my two weeks notice and moved back to the desert.

Another reason why I felt compelled to move back was that I was dating my current wife Juanita and I thought it was time to invest more in the relationship with her and her daughter, Ashley who I have grown to love as if she was my own. Actually, I see no difference. Ashley is my daughter.

Once in Arizona, I immediately landed a job working for a well-known communications company, and after one year they decided to relocate the company to the Philippines. Since there was no way I was moving to another country, I started applying for jobs and accepted a position at Compass Bank as the Assistant Vice president of Customer Service where I worked for ten years.

During that period, the Colorado Springs High School Sports Hall of Fame announced my 2006 induction. Being inducted was such an honor, and I was excited because I had a chance to travel back to

Colorado Springs where it all began. While there, I had an opportunity to visit my high school, (Widefield High), throw the coin toss at the high school football game, see some old friends, and talk to coaches who had taught me so much. I hadn't been back to Colorado Springs in over 25 years, so this was a great highlight at a much-needed time in my life.

Unfortunately my high came down quickly as I was informed that a Spanish bank purchased Compass Bank. With the transition, the bank decided to relocate the customer service department to Laredo Texas and offered me a Vice President position. An excellent opportunity, however, I would have had to relocate to Texas. Due to other obligations, and the fact that my beautiful baby, Darryana, was on the way, I had to decline the offer. Even though I was possibly going to be out of a job, my greatest joy was knowing that I had a baby girl on the way.

As I look back, from a professional standpoint, I regret not taking the offer to move to Laredo Texas as some opportunities only come knocking once. However, on the flip side, the birth of my daughter trumped everything.

I've learned in life that with patience and endurance, other doors open elsewhere that provide better opportunities so I was patient and hopeful that God would open a better door.

As I mentioned, I always felt a void in my life. I wanted to be involved in an organization helping others by giving back. In what capacity I had no idea, but that was a purpose that I had to fulfill. One evening, I attended a Dyslexia fundraising event hosted by a former NFL player friend.

During the event, I had a casual conversation with a guest by the name of Darius Perry. We discussed our lives, goals, hometowns, and more. He was a Dallas Cowboy fan from Texas and a retired army man who worked in the mental health field.

As we continued to talk, I realized we had many similarities. I'm a Cowboy fan and former player, I'm from Texas, and I'm an army brat.

Through our conversation, we discovered that we were both interested in hosting youth football camps, and speaking to kids about being good athletes, focusing on education, and being involved in the community.

Through many more conversations, and after meeting one of his counterparts from his job, Josh Jakubczak, we decided to establish a company and call it Sportmetric.

The company was created to host youth football camps for kids between seven to 17 years of age, stressing the importance of education and leadership, and strengthening philanthropic efforts by giving back to the community.

My job was to also speak about mental health, where we work with other organizations and non-profit organizations to help raise money for the cause. I fulfilled the missing void inside of me. It was a way for me to help others and give back through something I'm passionate about—football, education, and my community

Half Time

L et's take a break for a minute. You've read about my football career and how I flourished in track & field. You've traveled with me through school, and I've shared insight on concussion and my bout with depression.

This is a good time to stretch, get a glass of water or a cup of tea, and prepare yourself for what is about to take place during the second half. Some information will be a review, and for some, it will be enlightening.

I need you to hang on to every word and try to envision what I went through. Better yet, try to imagine yourself or a loved one going through my journey. The process surely puts things in perspective.

THIRD QUARTER: Working Through The Pain

During the process of launching SportMetric, Cox Communications hired me as a supervisor in the retention department. I managed a team of 25-plus representatives. While excelling and working hard in the company, meeting my sales goals and leading my team, my health was declining. My short-term memory became challenging.

However, this wasn't the first time my memory issue caused a problem. It happened a few times while I was working at Compass Bank and I would also have stints of dizziness for no apparent reason. On some occasions, while driving, I would have to pull over on the side of the road until the dizziness passed.

I was also experiencing headaches daily, and sometimes, a migraine would cause me to miss work. I reported this to my primary doctor. He ordered an MRI but could not determine anything. So I continued to fight through and keep working like a trained warrior. Hey! I'm a football player, and that's what I do. I work through the pain.

Fast forward to Cox Communications. As I attended meetings and training sessions and sometimes conducted them with my team, there were times I would forget the information that I had just learned. Not only did I have to make more of an effort to concentrate, but I also had to take more notes to ensure that I delegated effectively. The frustrating part is that this was information I knew, but the details were becoming fuzzy.

With all my brain fog I continued to work on Sportmetric goals as well—establishing youth camps, speaking at events and volunteering to help nonprofit organizations.

While at my 9 to 5, another issue I noticed was that pronouncing certain words became difficult. There were moments I'd find myself stuttering and not being able to put letters and words together. It caused me to make an extra effort to focus and to take my time when speaking as if it were a new skill I was learning. I could not understand why this was happening. However, I ignored the problems and kept working and managing my team to meet our goals. My two-part goal was to move up within Cox Communications and to make Sportmetric a premier nationally known company.

Time went by, and I tried to deal with my speech and memory issues on my own. What was I supposed to do? Since my doctor could not find anything wrong, I made the best of it and continued with my life. Although when I look back, I should have gotten a second opinion and pushed harder.

Ironically, in 2011, former retired NFL football players issued a lawsuit to the National Football League regarding concussions. This suit was regarding the NFL knowing and had reports, which stated that players with continuous head trauma or any concussions would most likely suffer severe neurological issues to include Parkinson's, Alzheimer's, Dementia and CTE. They never informed players that the helmets we used with the consistent head trauma would not be sufficient enough to protect the brain.

With all the confusing things going on in my life—mentally, physically and emotionally—I received the great news that lifted my spirits. The Arizona Leadership and Community Involvement presented me with an award for my community involvement. Winning the award allowed me the opportunity to throw the first pitch at the Arizona

Diamondback vs. San Francisco Giants baseball game. It was a fantastic experience and a great rush. It once again brought back many memories of me being on the field and playing ball.

That experience was a temporary high because when things calmed down, I still had to deal with my memory and speech issues that were still affecting my life negatively.

I continued working with these symptoms, and in 2015 my doctor suggested I see a Neurologist and Neurological Psychologist based on my symptoms. During each examination, both doctors determined I have beginning stages of dementia caused by continued head trauma.

While working at Cox Communications, I continued to stay busy, but I still wasn't feeling 100 percent. My job was demanding and my work hours were between 40 to 60 hours per week depending on requirements and projects.

Some of my job responsibilities were to attend meetings and training sessions as well as hire employees. I also had to meet sales goals, lead projects, manage my team on attendance and sales issues, and to work with other departments to help achieve and maintain objectives for the entire company, to name a few.

I have always been a high achiever and aspire to be the best at whatever I do. I wanted to move up in the company, and since the NFL offers tuition assistance plans, I decided I would go for a Ph.D. even with my health concerns. Some would say I was a bit ambitious. After researching universities and deciding what I would be interested in studying, I decided to attend the Grand Canyon University online program and pursue my Ph.D. in Education with an emphasis in Leadership.

The degree would allow me to enhance my ability to transform organizations for optimal success and growth. In a nutshell, the degree would prepare me to act as an agent of change in various types of organizations as an advanced professional position, or lead operations in an educational or corporate environment.

After a long day at work in September 2016, I started my first college course. If you aren't familiar with a Ph.D. program, it's an intense program where you are required to do a significant amount of research and writing. So, I'm working a full-time job, working part-time with my own company and attending college. What was I thinking?

My life became very stressful, and it became difficult to manage my time. I was up all hours of the night not getting much sleep, which was horrible because before attending school I probably averaged five hours of sleep nightly. Hence, sleep apnea, neurological conditions, dementia, and depression. Do you see how the dots are connecting?

I had to complete school assignments all week including weekends and meet deadlines for research papers. I had no time for myself, and became overwhelmed, tired, and frustrated because it was challenging to retain information.

I had to work hard to concentrate and take numerous amounts of notes that I would revisit to use for later assignments. I was still getting headaches, becoming moody and more irritable, and bouts of depression would appear.

I finally realized that I was not the man I used to be and that this was not going to work. For the first time in my adult life, I wanted to quit. Between my job at Cox, Sportmetric, my health issues, taking care of my family and the required demands of the Ph.D. program, there was no way I would be able to accomplish my goals.

As I started to evaluate my life, I realized that I had achieved a lot and that some things just weren't that important or worth jeopardizing my health. The Ph.D. program was rigorous and draining, and slowly falling from the top of my list. However, because I'm competitive, stubborn and love a challenge, I found new strength and convinced myself that I could win, so I pressed on.

Dementia! Really?

As I mentioned many times, I was having problems remembering and was experiencing headaches often. I first started noticing cognitive difficulties (I now know the term) in 2006. In 2010, I visited my doctor and told him about my problems with sleep, memory loss, and issues with focusing, and as I stated earlier, the outcome was inconclusive.

I decided to see a specialist so I could get to the bottom of this mystery. After being examined by a neurologist and neuropsychologist, my diagnosis was Neurocognitive Impairment with a severe decline in cognitive function—In layman's terms, my diagnosis was early-stage dementia.

Dementia refers to a group of symptoms that affect memory, thinking, and social skills severely enough to interfere with daily functioning. It is not a specific disease, but a group of symptoms caused by various diseases and conditions. No one test can determine if an individual has dementia. Dementia does not have a cure, and no treatment can entirely halt its progression.

Alzheimer's is the most common type of dementia, accounting for 60 to 80-percent of cases. Vascular dementia, previously known as post-stroke dementia, is the second most common type of dementia, accounting for 10-percent of cases, according to Active Beat.

Doctors diagnose dementia based on careful medical history, a physical examination, laboratory tests, and the characteristic changes in thinking, day-to-day function, and behavior associated with each type.

They can determine that a person has dementia with a high level of certainty. However, it's harder to determine the exact nature of dementia because the symptoms and brain changes of different dementias can overlap. In some cases, a doctor may diagnose "dementia" and not specify a type.

The characteristic change I noticed in myself is day-to-day thinking. Some days I have to force myself to focus, and I struggle to retain information. My family noticed cognitive changes such as directional abilities, following my routine, and occasionally missing exits on the freeway and forgetting my intended destination. I've also lost my car in parking lots many times. Another example is when grocery shopping, I would have a list but forgot I had it and would forget to buy things.

Let's talk about my emotional being. My mood swings are always up and down, I have symptoms of sadness and low motivation and in many cases, not realizing it, I isolate myself.

For the most part, I'm confident and energetic, and I engage in physical activities. I have periods of aggressive behavior, and I would have rare moments of suicidal intent but would snap out of it quickly.

As always I reported this to my primary care physician. Sleep or lack thereof is another issue I've dealt with consistently.

In 2015, I underwent a sleep study that revealed I had sleep apnea. Sleep apnea, a common disorder in athletes, is a disorder characterized by pauses in breathing or periods of shallow breathing during sleep. I sometimes wake up in the middle of the night choking, and a few times my wife witnessed that I stopped breathing. With sleep apnea, a CPAP (continuous positive airway pressure) is used to help with breathing.

Finding the right CPAP mask that I felt comfortable with and that would match my sleeping pattern was challenging. I tend to sleep on my back and my side and sometimes on my stomach, so it made it extremely difficult to get a good night's rest with it on my face.

Fortunately, a dentist I met created and was approved for a specific type of dental device or mouth guard to wear at night. The guard opens the mouth by bringing the mandible forward. I was authorized to wear the mouth guard. It minimized my snoring and helped me maintain proper airflow through my mouth so I could continue to breathe.

To evaluate the cause of my early-stage dementia, as I stated earlier, I sustained my first concussion in the fifth grade along with daily head trauma through contact football. Followed by three years of junior high school with daily head trauma through contact football and another three years of high school football with another concussion and daily head trauma.

Once in college, I experienced yet another concussion with daily head trauma, and finally four years in the NFL, one year in the CFL and another year in the NFL World League with daily head trauma, and my share of several concussions. If I combine all the hits to my head, that totals to about fifteen years of head trauma from contact football. As a result of this constant head trauma, I have sustained some symptoms that undoubtedly led to dementia.

So what are my symptoms? Memory loss; having trouble with communicating and pronouncing certain words; inability to focus and pay attention; reasoning and judgment; visual perception; problems with short-term memory; issues with keeping track of things; paying bills; planning and preparing meals; remembering appointments; and traveling back to my neighborhood depending on what direction I'm coming from.

Declining: inability to recall a short-term memory or recent events such as what I did yesterday or last week. However, suddenly a keen ability to remember specifics from the past will occur.

Listed below are the ten common symptoms of dementia, according to Activebeat.co:

- Motor function: lose the physical ability to perform routine tasks like go to the washroom, drive to your grocery store, operate the stove and need 24-hour care for your safety.
- Disorientation: this may cause you to become confused and lost when out on your own, and you may not be able to remember where they are, or how you got there, or how and where to return home. At times you may gradually start to forget familiar people, places, facts, the time of day, the year, or other pertinent facts.
- Behavioral changes: Personality changes that may include becoming cranky when you were always easy going or just being inappropriate in public.
- Paranoia: suspicious of others and losing control.
- Disorganization: Difficulty with planning and organizing a person may suddenly have difficulty planning their grocery shopping or finding their glasses that they always put in the same location.
- Agitation: frustration over the inability to carry out simple tasks, the inability to communicate, fatigue, or fear as "control" such as a driver's license or a home being taken away.
- Hallucinations: visual, seeing things that aren't there or hearing noises that aren't there such as the belief that a person is out to get them without reason. Having delusions is characterized as believing in false things (i.e., people, memories, details, and events). However, hallucinations are different. When suffering a hallucination, an individual has a false perception--a false perception of an event, objects, or person that's sensory.

- Sexual Actions: suddenly become sexual without awareness that their actions are inappropriate—for instance, removing clothing, exposing oneself in public, or touching and saying tasteless things to strangers and caregivers.
- Cognitive Decline: The inability to reason or a decline in cognitive functions—such as thinking, learning, reading and retaining information, problem-solving, language and speech.

Also resulting in trouble with memory, the performance of mundane daily tasks, losing objects, the inability to use the right word, forgetting names or people, and trouble with planning, remember dates, and organizational skills.

According to alz.org, damaged brain cells cause dementia. This damage affects the ability of the brain cells to communicate with each other. When brain cells do not interact with each other, thinking, behavior, and feelings are affected. The brain has many distinct regions; each region is responsible for different functions like memory, judgment, and movement. When cells in a particular area are damaged, that region cannot carry what it's responsible for holding.

Most changes in the brain that cause dementia are permanent and can worsen over time or as you get older. Although there is no specific type of treatment to help prevent dementia, in most cases, there are medications to help improve the condition.

There have been doctors who have told me the best way is to work my brain and keep it active such as doing crossword puzzles for example that forces your brain cells to push themselves to work.

Also, smoking is not recommended; maintaining your blood pressure, blood sugar, and cholesterol at the recommended levels and exercising is imperative. This lifestyle helps the brain cells due to increased blood oxygen flow to the brain. A healthy diet and a healthy heart is also a significant benefit. A suggestion is a diet that contains less red meat, but whole grains, fruits, vegetables, fish shellfish, nuts, and olive oil.

It's a known fact that as we age, our risk of dementia increases. According to activebeat.org, by the age of 85 almost 35-percent of those in this age group experience this degenerative disorder that causes gradually and worsening memory loss and mental skills.

Nearly 30 percent of former NFL players will develop brain conditions like Alzheimer's or a form of dementia, according to a report released by the NFL and the NFL Players' Association. That's 3 in 10 former NFL football players who will get Alzheimer's or Dementia. However, not everyone will experience all of the symptoms mentioned.

For example, there have been times when my daughter, Darryana and I have been in a store, and I'll ask a salesperson to point me in the direction of a particular product. According to my daughter, I would become upset when I felt the salesperson was not answering my question in detail, but I had no idea that I exploded until my daughter would ask if I was okay.

She would then explain that I was irritable and acting upset towards the salesperson for no reason. She would say, "Daddy your tone changed, and you weren't smiling. You weren't the same person you were when we walked in the store." Having my daughter notice the sudden change in my behavior for no reason at all is concerning.

I recall my wife asking me to do something as minor as rake the leaves in the yard, take out the trash or even pick up something from the grocery store on my way home from work. I'd agree to do it but, when she asked later about her request, I had no recollection of her asking.

Episodes of forgetfulness happen occasionally and eventually caused hostility in my marriage. If you're in a relationship, married, or have friends who are suffering from any level of dementia you have to buckle up and get ready for the ride. It's not easy, but if you equip yourself with information, try to be more understanding and patient, research the symptoms, become an advocate with your loved one for their health, and by all means be more selfless, it will undoubtedly help the situation.

Rather than wanting to give others our time and our help, most tend to worry about their wants and needs. Whether you're a wife, husband, brother, sister, friend or parent, you must practice selflessness and patience. You have to have empathy for others and put yourself in their shoes. Is it going to be hard? Yes. However, if you love the person enough, you'll learn how to adjust and provide a caring environment.

A perfect bible scripture about selflessness is in 1 Peter 3:8—"Finally, all of you, have unity of mind, sympathy, brotherly love, a tender heart, and a humble mind." It takes an exceptional individual to endure patience and show love, compassion, acceptance, and understanding when helping someone throughout an illness. By working together, you can achieve the overall long-term goal—and that is to win.

To win or even slow down the process of full-blown dementia, I need to be an advocate for my health. In my search for answers, I read an article by betternutrition.com entitled, "10 Causes of Possibly Reversible Dementia" where the author, Vera Tweed, uncovers ten underlying issues that may be at the root of dementia.

I've listed seven that caught my eye:

1. Toxins have been shown to kill brain cells. They damage the lining of our gut, create inflammation, impair immune function, and disrupt hormones, all of which can contribute to brain fog or dementia. Pesticides and herbicides are toxins that are relatively simple to avoid if you eat organic food.

2. Diabetes is known to increase the risk of dementia, but even slightly elevated blood sugar in healthy people increases risk. Insulin resistance, where blood glucose cannot be utilized for energy, is also linked to dementia. Avoiding high-starch,

high-sugar foods, and drinks can help prevent and reverse the condition.

3. Too little sleep or lack thereof adds a higher risk for dementia. Allowing enough time and, if necessary, taking supplements such as 5-HTP, melatonin, magnesium, or tart cherry juice, can help improve sleep.

4. Deficiencies of vitamins B1 and B12 are triggers of dementia symptoms. B1, depleted by alcohol and poorly absorbed by gluten-sensitive people, is essential for blood sugar to be used as energy in the brain, and a deficiency leads to the death of brain cells. B12 becomes harder to absorb, as people get older, and is an essential component of myelin, a protective coating on brain cells. Deficiencies in vitamin B6 and folic acid can also contribute to dementia symptoms. All of these B vitamins can be found in B complex or multivitamin formulas, or as individual supplements.

5. Studies found that hearing loss increases the risk for dementia and that correcting hearing problems stop or slows down mental decline.

6. Studies show that exercise can improve memory, speed up thinking, and improve focus. The latest guidelines from the American Academy of Neurology recommend brisk walking, jogging, or other activities that get your heart pumping, at least twice weekly, for a total of 150 minutes per week. Weight training, while necessary for preserving muscle, hasn't been shown to protect against dementia.

7. Social inactivity leads to cognitive impairments. Making a habit of spending time with friends, visiting relatives, and going to parties, restaurants, and other events lower the odds of dementia, according to a study.

I'm no doctor, and I know the odds of my early-stage dementia disappearing is entirely up to God, but I'm willing to do my part to at least slow down the process, and altering my lifestyle to incorporate healthy eating is a start.

FOURTH QUARTER:
My Fight to Live

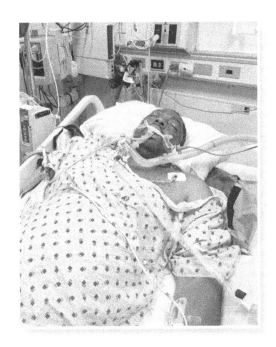

I n 2016 my medical history showed obstructive sleep apnea and multiple concussions with early dementia, with bouts of depression—my usual state of health. However, one day in late September 2016, I began to develop recurrent mild headaches and dark urine for approximately one week. I thought it was the stress from work and school and

I needed to rest, so my family and I went on vacation to Oceanside, California.

On the first day of vacation, I felt okay. We spent time on the beach then decided to have lunch at a restaurant. While eating lunch my left arm became numb, my speech became slurred, and I was not able to hold a complete conversation. My family started asking me questions, but I was unable to answer them intelligently and was unable to pronounce certain words. This feeling was very familiar because I had bouts with confusion and articulating words months before this happened.

I somehow got through lunch, and when I could not write my name on the credit card receipt, my wife asked me if I was okay. At that moment I wasn't sure, and I said, "I don't know, I'm not feeling well." I felt as if I was dozing off.

My wife called 911 immediately and the ambulance arrived fast. They began to take my vital signs and quickly determined that I needed to get to the hospital. I was placed on a gurney, put in the ambulance, and on my way to Tri-City Medical Center in Oceanside, CA.

Three hundred seventy-five miles from home and out of all the hospitals in Oceanside, California I happened to be within a few miles of one that specializes in neurological conditions. A coincidence? I think not. The doctors at Tri City Medical Center diagnosed me very fast.

I acquired Thrombotic thrombocytopenic purport (TTP) and atypical hemolytic uremic syndrome (aHUS). A double whammy!

Time Out!

In sports, a timeout is a halt in the play that allows the coaches of either team to communicate with the team to determine strategy or inspire morale, and inform as well as to stop the game clock.

The NFL limits the number of timeouts that a team can call. Each team is allowed to call three timeouts per half. This is my timeout to prepare you for what's to come.

It took me some time to understand my illness or even pronounce it so for you to get it all in one sitting is going to take concentration.

As you proceed, you may come across terms that may be foreign to you but very important in understanding my journey and the importance of sharing.

Thrombotic Thrombocytopenic Purport (TTP)

I t's time to dissect the illness that threatened my life. TTP is a severe and life-threatening autoimmune blood disease. It is a medical emergency that 10-20% of acute patients die from despite currently available treatments. TTP is a lifelong condition, and many people who suffer from this will experience further episodes or relapses after the initial diagnoses.

In TTP, blood clots form in small blood vessels throughout the body. The clots can limit or block the flow of oxygen-rich blood to the body's organs, such as the brain, kidneys, and heart. As a result, serious health problems can develop.

Ironically, head injuries can lead immune-system brain cells to go on "high alert" and overreact to later immune challenges by becoming excessively inflammatory.

A few key points:

- TTP is an ultra-rare and potentially life-threatening condition
- 30%-50% of patients will experience multiple episodes of TTP (called relapses) after their initial diagnosis

- It occurs when the ADAMTS13 enzyme does not function as it should, leading to small blood clots in the blood vessels, low platelet counts and destruction of red blood cells
- What causes the body to start producing antibodies against ADAMTS13 in acquired TTP is unknown
- Patients with TTP may experience a wide variety of symptoms, including fever, fatigue, headache, confusion and bruises or dots on the skin
- There are two main types of TTP – inherited TTP and acquired TTP

I acquired TTP. I wasn't born with it (inherited) but instead developed it later in life. In TTP, the body's immune system starts producing antibodies that stop ADAMTS13 from working. The ADAMTS13 gene provides instructions for making an enzyme that is involved in blood clotting.

After an injury, clots usually protect the body by sealing off damaged blood vessels and preventing further blood loss. Okay, okay, I know you're saying to yourself, "What in the world is ADAMTS13?" It's a lot to digest so I'll give it to you according to Wikipedia.

The ADAMTS13 enzyme processes a large protein called the von Willebrand factor, which also plays a role in clot formation. The unprocessed form of von Willebrand factor interacts easily with cell fragments called platelets, which circulate in the bloodstream and are essential for blood clotting.

TTP Symptoms

In my research, I found that each TTP patient is different and that they may experience a wide range of symptoms because the entire body is affected. Many people, like me, may initially experience general, symptoms such as fever or flu-like symptoms. However, the different processes generally lead to two main types of symptoms—symptoms caused by bleeding and symptoms caused by the formation of blood clots.

Symptoms of TTP caused by bleeding include:

- Bleeding from the gums or nose, which may be caused by thrombocytopenia
- Purple bruises on the skin called purpura and red or purple dots on the skin called petechiae, which are caused by bleeding under the skin

Symptoms caused by the formation of blood clots include:

- Headaches, confusion & disturbed vision, which may be caused by blood clots blocking the flow of blood to the brain
- Chest pain, which may be caused by blood clots blocking the flow of blood to the heart
- Fatigue, jaundice (a yellowing of the skin and eyes) & dark urine that may be caused by hemolytic anemia

- Kidney problems, which may be caused by blood clots blocking the flow of blood to the kidney

While in the ambulance the EMTs began to work on me persistently. I told them that I was feeling extraordinarily nauseous so they gave me medication. At that point, I blacked out. When I woke, I was told that the EMTs immediately implemented stroke workup (thank God it was negative) because I was showing stroke symptoms. The workup included to CT head scan, CT angiogram head, and neck scan, and an MRI of the brain. CT is short for computerized tomography. Tomograpy is a method of producing a three-dimensional image of the human body.

The EMT's implemented stroke workup because I was showing symptoms of a stroke.

TTP may be expected as the underlying cause of stroke if there is a prior history of TTP. I had no previous history of TTP and no family medical history of stroke. However, I had stroke-like symptoms to include numbness in left arm—when my family and I were at the restaurant I tried to raise my arm or grip the ink pen to sign the credit card bill but I could not. My speech slurred, I wasn't responsive to questions, and I had difficulty in vision in both eyes, sudden severe headache, and felt as if I was going to doze off.

The Initial labs were significant for hemoglobin of 11 as well as platelets of 11 and acute kidney injury with a creatinine level of 1.75mg. Normal creatinine serum blood levels are 0.6 to 1.2 mg/dl. Creatine is an amino acid located mostly in your body's muscles, as well as in the brain.

The body's liver, pancreas, and kidneys also make creatine. Elevated creatinine level signifies impaired kidney function or kidney disease. Thank God the doctors at the hospital were able to lower my level.

However, to date, my current doctors check my kidneys periodically to ensure normalcy and to detect any change.

Normal Hemoglobin levels in an adult male are 14 to 18 gm/dL, and normal platelet counts range from 150,000 - 400,000 per mm3 of blood. Any time your platelet count drops below 50,000 per mm3 you are considered to be at increased risk for bleeding. In a nutshell, my body was in a dangerous state.

Finally, after hematology (the study of the cause, prognosis, treatment, and prevention of diseases related to blood) and nephrology (Nephrology concerns the diagnosis and treatment of kidney diseases) services were consulted, the diagnosis was an acquired thrombotic thrombocytopenic purpura (TTP).

Because acquired TTP is an uncommon blood disease and autoimmune disorder that is life threatening, it requires prompt diagnosis and initiation of therapeutic plasma exchange or plasmapheresis to improve patient survival. In many cases, plasmapheresis is used to remove the antibodies that inhibit the ADAMTS13 protease and also add back the functional ADAMTS13 protein.

In this process blood is removed by a machine from the affected individual, blood cells are separated from plasma, the patient's plasma is replaced with healthy plasma, and the blood is then returned to the patient by the machine.

I give credit to the doctors at Tri-City for acting fast. However, the ultimate credit goes to God for placing me in the right place at the right time. Jeremiah 29:11 NLT states, "For I know the plans I have for you," says the LORD. "They are plans for good and not for disaster, to give you a future and a hope…"

God will use His perfect timing, and whatever means necessary to ensure that we are fulfilling his ultimate plans for us. In my case, He placed the restaurant in precisely the right place and the EMT drivers at the right time for my benefit.

My ADAM TS-13 level came back with activity less than five. Measurement of ADAM TS-13 activity is the most commonly used test in the workup of suspected TTP, and I had schistocytes on peripheral smear.

Schistocytes are circulating red blood cell fragments. Detection of this is an essential clue for the diagnosis of TTP. A blood smear is a blood test used to look for abnormalities in blood cells. The blood cells that the test focuses on are red cells, which carry oxygen throughout your body, white cells, which help your body fight infections and other inflammatory diseases.

With the results from all the tests, I stated that the doctors immediately started me on therapeutic plasma exchange or plasmapheresis. However, during the process, I had a seizure and slipped into a coma. Hold tight. I'll get to the coma in a bit.

The doctors had to continue examining me for any neurological damage, and because of this it resulted in an inability to protect my airway, so I was intubated to maintain an open airway and immediately transferred to the ICU.

As days passed, my symptoms improved with daily plasma exchange, though I continued to have low platelets and high LDH. LDH is an enzyme, or catalyst, found in many different tissues in your body. These include your red blood cells, skeletal muscles, kidneys, brain, and lungs. When your LDH rises, it means that tissues may have been damaged or are diseased.

According to the Department of Biostatistics & Epidemiology, College of Public Health, OUHSC, some patients with TTP still, die.

In my research I learned that most patients with TTP died because they never had a chance for effective treatment; patients given plasma exchange treatments have almost always survived. Survival is even more likely now than it was only ten years ago, because of the more frequent use of steroids – sometimes in very high doses – and also rituximab when the initial response to PEX is not sufficient.

Today, the expected survival rate is over 90%. However, this expectation is for patients who are diagnosed promptly and treated appropriately.

If the doctors had not diagnosed me with TTP and immediately started treating me with Plasma Exchange, I would have died. I'm so thankful for their diligent work, and I praise God for allowing them to not give up on me.

To quote the late evangelist, Billy Graham, "God spared you for a purpose, and the most important thing you can do is to seek that purpose and dedicate your life to it. You aren't here by chance, nor are you here to live for yourself without any thought of God. God made you, and life's greatest joy comes from knowing Him and living for Him every day."

I know God spared me and that I had to do better. Be better, and give him praise with every opportunity.

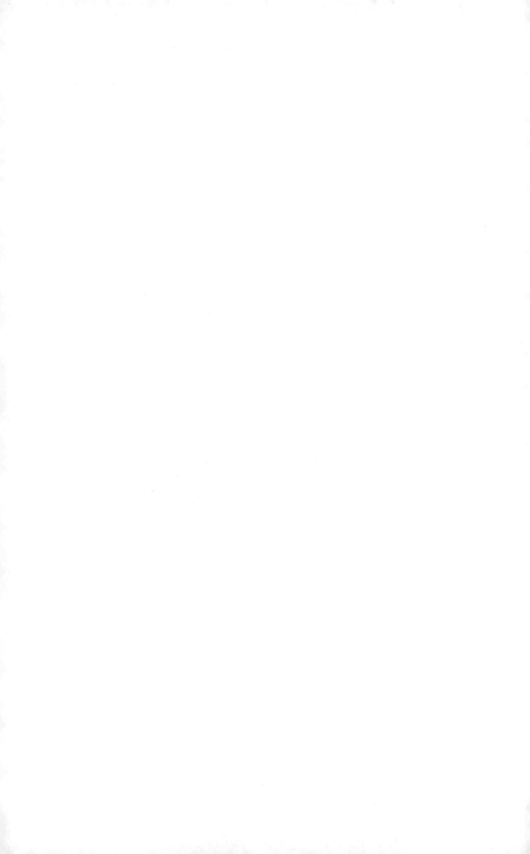

Atypical HUS or Thrombotic Thrombocytopenic Purpura?

As an advocate for my health, I'm always researching to find a better understanding of my complex illnesses that doctors have explained to me for the past two years yet still have me perplexed at times.

The aHUS alliance website described my experience and understanding perfectly, "vague symptoms that quickly become urgent, medical symptoms that are common to many different diagnoses, a syndrome few doctors have experience treating, and a sporadic and complex disease that can affect multiple organs and body systems."

The website also helped me understand why Atypical Hemolytic Uremic Syndrome (aHUS) and Thrombotic Thrombocytopenic Purpura (TTP) are hard to decipher.

Here's the difference. For both aHUS and TTP, an essential characteristic is the tiny clots (thrombotic microangiopathy or TMA) that can form throughout the body, in addition to other common features such as red blood cell destruction, low platelet counts, and kidney injury.

Diagnosis of TTP involves an ADAMTS13 test (assay) to determine its activity percent, with low results noted in about 80% of patients with thrombotic thrombocytopenic purpura (TTP).

Sometimes aHUS patients have a partial ADAMTS13 deficiency, further emphasizing that atypical HUS is often a 'diagnosis of exclusion' as doctors rule out other diseases until the only diagnosis left is aHUS.

Yeah, yeah I know this is quite confusing, but the information I'm giving you could help you or someone you love. With a blink of an eye, my illnesses were a game changer, and I wish I had been equipped with the knowledge beforehand. So, hang in there while I continue my lesson.

Atypical Hemolytic Uremic Syndrome

Now that I've explained TTP lets breakdown atypical hemolytic uremic syndrome (aHUS), yet another disease and a piece of my medical puzzle. First of all, TTP and aHUS are two clinically similar disorders and are difficult to distinguish. Yikes!

aHUS is a rare, life-threatening, genetic disease that can damage vital organs such as the kidneys, heart, and brain. In patients with aHUS, blood clots form in small blood vessels throughout the body, a process known as systemic thrombotic microangiopathy, or TMA, a severe but rare medical disease.

It is a pattern of damage that can occur in the smallest blood vessels inside many of the body's vital organs – most commonly the kidney and brain. I had a blood vessel problem.

According to rarediseases.org, Atypical hemolytic uremic syndrome (aHUS) is characterized by low levels of circulating red blood cells due to their destruction (hemolytic anemia), low platelet count (thrombocytopenia) due to their consumption and inability of the kidneys to process waste products from the blood and excrete them into the urine (acute kidney failure), a condition known as uremia.

The terminology surrounding this disorder can be confusing. aHUS is considered a form of thrombotic microangiopathy (TMA). TMA is broken down into two primary types – thrombotic thrombocytopenia purpura and hemolytic uremic syndrome.

I learned that the onset of aHUS ranges from before birth (prenatally) to adulthood. Amid everything, I found out that I was born with aHUS, but it wasn't triggered until I acquired TTP. Who knew?

Here's another piece of the puzzle. Soliris, the medication that I've taken consistently for at least 18 months, is the first and only therapy approved for the treatment of atypical hemolytic uremic syndrome (aHUS) that improves platelet and red blood cell counts. It may also reverse acute kidney injury and prevent kidney failure if taken soon enough.

It all started to make sense. The plasmapheresis for TTP in conjunction with other drugs that suppress my immune system (immunosuppressive therapy) and improve platelet and red blood cell counts was to treat both diseases simultaneously. Some were used to help my brain and heart, and others to support my kidney. Whew! I should apply for medical school.

aHUS Symptoms

A ccording to ahussource.com, people with aHUS are at constant risk of sudden, catastrophic, and life-threatening symptoms and complications. As the disease continues to damage small blood vessels, vital organs can fail to work, either suddenly or over time.

Symptoms of aHUS most often include:

- Nausea and vomiting
- Confusion
- Shortness of breath
- Fatigue
- Anemia (low red blood cell/platelet count in the blood)
- Thrombocytopenia (low platelet count in the blood)
- Kidney (renal) symptoms, including kidney damage, kidney failure or end-stage renal disease (i.e., damage requiring chronic dialysis)

The symptoms described above may continue to worsen during active episodes or attacks. In some cases, severe, non-kidney related symptoms present themselves right away, and in others, symptoms do not occur until later.

Symptoms can include:

- Stroke
- Gastrointestinal problems including severe stomach pain
- Inflamed colon
- Blood vessel damage
- Heart attacks
- Neurological issues including seizures

The Brain, Heart, Kidneys and Nervous System

A HUS and TTP affect various organs, including the brain, heart, kidneys, lungs, and gastrointestinal systems. With aHUS and TTP it's hard to say what in the body is affected first, last or not at all. If the brain is the central computer that controls all bodily functions, then the nervous system is like a network that relays messages back and forth from the brain to different parts of the body.

So, if one is not functioning correctly, it creates an unbalanced system.

The brain controls what you think and feel, how you learn and remember, and the way you move and talk, the beating of your heart, the digestion of your food, and even the amount of stress you feel.

A part of the peripheral nervous system called the autonomic nervous system is responsible for controlling many of the body processes like breathing, digesting, sweating, and chills. This nervous system has two parts: the sympathetic and the parasympathetic nervous systems.

The sympathetic nervous system prepares the body for sudden stress, like bracing yourself for a car accident about to happen. The sympathetic nervous system makes the heart beat faster by sending blood more quickly to the different body parts that might need it. It also causes the adrenal glands at the top of the kidneys to release adrenaline, a hormone that helps give extra power to the muscles to move quickly, if needed. (Kidshealth.org).

The brain is a muscle and indeed the central computer that controls all body functions. So think about how my body was functioning due to acquiring TTP and aHUS. Everything was out of whack. My system was under attack, and it wasn't fun.

The Mystery of the Mind: Comatose

Speaking of the brain, let's discuss my coma experience. I always wondered if a person in a coma could hear or even understand what people were saying to them or what doctors were discussing in their hospital room.

Many stories I've read about former patients who reveal what it felt like to be in a coma usually had something to do with a dream that was brought on by conversations around or in their room.

One story I read was about a guy who awoke from a coma terrified because his leg was either amputated or was going to be amputated. It took him three days to ask the doctors and his parents about his leg. When he did, they all looked at him like he was crazy. It was at that moment he found out that in the next room over, there was a gentleman who had diabetes and they were going to amputate his leg.

He heard the conversation when he was in the coma and assumed they were talking about him. He had surgery to fix his collapsed right lung, no amputations.

My experience was different. Although I had a dream, I didn't hear nurses or doctors. It was darkness and calmness like I was sleeping but searching for something. It was a dream about my life and what I needed to do differently to become a better person. I knew I needed a better relationship with God before the coma, so I'm sure this was the last thing on my mind before I slipped into a coma.

My dream magnified my thoughts and concerns. I was talking to God more, and I believe he instilled something in me because now, more than ever I get extra emotional when I observe certain things or events with people. I think God softened my heart and made me more sympathetic.

As a football player, I'm trained to endure pain and hide my feelings; however, this experience has indeed changed my way of thinking.

While I was in a coma, I heard my wife talk to me when she visited. I also heard one of my best friends and college football teammates, Stein Koss, speak to me firmly in my ear. He said, "D.C. this is Stein; please fight through this I know you can do this. Love you brother." I remember responding to him in my mind saying, "Yes, I will fight."

Eventually, I awoke. I explain this as if I woke up immediately after Stein whispered in my ear, but honestly, I don't know how much time passed before I opened my eyes.

Yes, I woke up but the question is, "Who woke me up?" The last thing I heard while in a coma was a voice saying "Get Up!" I woke up out of the coma and was told by my nurse, I began ripping wires off of my body and proceeded to walk out of my hospital room as if I had somewhere to go.

The doctors, nurses and some of the staff had to restrain me in fear of me causing more damage to myself. The nurse said this was the first time she had ever witnessed anything like that in all her years working with comatose patients.

Later, once I had my wits and thought about it, I realized that the voice I heard was God.

Proverbs 16:20 states, "Those who listen to instruction will prosper; those who trust the Lord will be joyful." There's no other explanation as to whom I heard and why I did what I did. God woke me up, and because my body was so still and at peace, I was able to hear Him and follow instructions.

However, it's deeper than that. I could have died in the hospital, but God let me live. 2 Peter: 3 states, "The Lord isn't being slow about his promise, as some people think. No, he is being patient for your sake. He does not want anyone to be destroyed, but wants everyone to repent." This incredible out of body experience was my chance to get my life right.

I'm sure many things happened while I was unconscious and that many of my dreams may come back to me one day, but it's the strangest thing being in a coma. People say it's like deep sleep.

In the article, 'What Exactly is a Coma and What Happens to You When You're in One?' in Braincharm.com, the writer states, "Some people who have been in comas have reported vivid dreams and hallucinations. Also, in some cases, what's going on around the comatose person gets incorporated into these dreams."

Waking up from a coma is scary. It's confusing. It feels nothing like actual sleep. I now see why doctors urge family and friends to talk to their loved ones who are in a coma because they could potentially hear you. I am a believer and a testament to this, and I thank God for my experience.

Platelets and Their Function

efore I continue, I need to define platelets and their functions. Platelets are tiny blood cells that help your body form clots to stop bleeding. If one of your blood vessels gets damaged, it sends out signals that are picked up by platelets. The platelets then rush to the damaged area and form a plug, or clot, to repair the damage.

The process of spreading across the surface of a damaged blood vessel to stop bleeding is called adhesion. Because when platelets get to the site of the injury, they grow sticky tentacles that help them adhere. They also send out chemical signals to attract more platelets to pile onto the clot in a process called aggregation.

Platelets are produced in the bone marrow along with white and red blood cells. Your bone marrow is the spongy center inside your bones. Another name for platelets is thrombocytes. Healthcare providers usually call a clot a thrombus. Once platelets are made and circulated into your bloodstream, they live for eight to ten days. A normal platelet count is 150,000 to 450,000 platelets per microliter of blood.

A risk for spontaneous bleeding develops if a platelet count falls below 10,000 to 20,000. When the platelet count is less than 50,000, bleeding is likely to be more severe if an individual is cut or bruised. When diagnosed with TTP my platelet count was 11,000. Whoa!

I initially had a temporary right Internal Jugular dialysis catheter placed in my right chest that later converted to a tunneled catheter, that I was using without difficulty. A tunneled central line is a catheter (a thin tube) placed in a vein for long-term use.

A tunneled catheter is used when someone needs intravenous (IV) access so they can receive fluids, transfusions, or drugs for an extended period (generally longer than three months), or when there is a need for many blood draws for lab tests.

I was getting Plasma Apheresis treatments daily to get my platelet count normal. I was also treated with steroids and was on methylprednisolone 100 mg q.8h. I was placed on rituximab with the first dose taken on October 1, 2016, and was scheduled to receive doses of 900 mg three times, seven days apart, with the next dose due on, October 28, 2016.

My symptoms improved with treatment, and I had no further seizures and no current neurologic deficits.

I also sustained memory loss and speech complications. I was like a little kid. I didn't have any taste buds, and the food served was horrible. Nobody likes hospital food, but this was different. I had absolutely no taste buds. I worked with a speech therapist to help me learn to speak and pronounce words as well. It was as if I was starting over with everything. I even had a physical therapist to teach me how to walk again.

I underwent all those different treatments every day, and it paid off because I started getting better and was able to speak and have complete conversations, and I was soon able to stand up and walk with a walker. Mr. "Cool" Clack lacked swag, but hey, you have to crawl before you walk.

Even though I was not able to walk on my own, it was a start and showed improvement. Parts of my memory started to come back but not everything.

After being in the hospital for about three weeks, I requested a transfer to Mayo Clinic because I lived in the Phoenix, AZ area and wanted to be closer to home, and also because the Mayo Clinic experts are some of the best in the world.

In the U.S. News & World Report rankings of top hospitals, Mayo Clinic consistently ranks among the top hospitals in the nation. Their highly specialized experts are more experienced in treating rare and complex conditions and 88% of patients who came to Mayo Clinic for a second opinion received a new or refined diagnosis.

Once the doctors approved my transport from Oceanside, California to Phoenix, Arizona I learned that my transportation options were by plane or ambulance. My doctor informed me that it wasn't a good idea to travel by plane because I would need a medical person to be with me in the event I had a relapse.

My options were abruptly canceled due to complications with my insurance. They stated because this was not a life-threatening situation they would not cover the transfer. Uh, hello! How about doing your research? My doctors and caseworker informed the insurance company that my illness was a life and death matter, but of course, they did not understand or try to understand the urgency.

My caseworker even sent them a break down of the cost of how it would cost less for the insurance company if I were back in Arizona. So, one would think it would be a no-brainer if they could save money, but they didn't budge. They denied my claim. That meant I had to find a private ambulance company and pay out-of-pocket for the transfer.

The transport included two EMT's and my mom who was not leaving my side. We drove from Oceanside, CA to Phoenix, AZ, and throughout the five-hour-drive, I had no complications. Thank God.

To offset the ambulance fee, my oldest daughter Ashley took it upon herself to start a GoFundMe® campaign that raised a nice amount of money. I'm grateful for Ashley and to everyone who donated to my cause. It was a blessing at such a crucial time.

My Medical Journey: Mayo Clinic

E ven though the Mayo Clinic allows patients to look up their lab results, doctor's notes and medical history on the hospital portal, I decided to keep a personal journal so that I could better understand what was going on with my body.

On October 27, 2016, the Mayo Clinic admitted me. On arrival, I was tachycardic (tachy·car·dia | \ ˌta-ki-ˈkär-dē-ə)

Which meant I had a fast resting heart rate but otherwise stable. I was currently feeling better with my only symptom being mild residual swelling and tingling of my right upper leg. I had some scattered bruising over my bilateral upper extremities at the site of previous blood draws, but I didn't have any prior history with easy bleeding or bruising. Nor did I have any further headaches or chest pain, dyspnea, abdominal pain, nausea, vomiting, or diarrhea. Internal Medicine Service admitted me for additional management.

The Mayo Clinic had all my administration paperwork completed, and my room was ready. It was a smooth transition with wonderful staff giving me a warm welcome. I felt I was in great hands.

On October 28, 2016, one day before my birthday, I met with my transfusion medicine doctor to go over my TTP assessment plan. She explained to me in full detail what their goal was and made sure I understood the details of my illness, as well as what their plan was to tackle my disease. The objective was to get my platelet count steady at or above 150k.

My doctor answered all my questions in detail, but what I liked most was that even though my case was rare and extremely new—most people either have aHUS or TTP but rarely do they have both together—the doctor and her team were confident that they would get results. I believed this because my doctor was very determined throughout my case, and the Mayo Clinic in Phoenix is a teaching hospital.

In my opinion, teaching hospitals often offer better care and more cutting-edge treatment than non-teaching hospitals. They have a responsibility to incorporate the latest techniques and medical advances into their treatments because they are training up-and-coming doctors. That was a win-win for me because of my challenging case. Having student doctors around keeps doctors on their toes because the students are always asking challenging questions.

Take the TV show "Greys Anatomy" for example. When the doctors make their rounds visiting the patient's rooms, they usually have at least five student doctors with them who ask a bunch of questions, and it's the doctor's job to ensure that their answers are accurate because one day the students will be practicing medicine solo.

If the doctor makes a mistake in feeding information to the student, and the student applies what they learned, it could be a dangerous situation. So, despite everything I was going through, I was confident and grateful to be at the Mayo Clinic. Happy Birthday to me!

After meeting with my doctors and receiving treatment, my platelets improved to 129K, and the doctors planned to do daily TPE (therapeutic plasma exchange) for three days until my platelet count normalized at which point they would taper. The TPE procedure can last between one to three hours and some people, depending on the illness, may need as many as five treatments per week. I was patient but also anxious to see how I would improve with the procedure.

On November 3, 2016, I was a bit discouraged. Remember the doctors informed me not to be surprised if my platelet count dropped? My platelets decreased to 106K. Not unexpected given the refractory nature of my course thus far.

The doctors recommended keeping me in the hospital until we started to see progress towards halting the TMA process. With the TMA process, my platelet counts would improve in the setting of active TMA because they are supplying me with a temporary source of ADAMTS13 enzyme from donor plasma during the TPE.

Now, remember, the ADAMTS13 gene provides instructions for making an enzyme that is involved in blood clotting. The enzyme processes a large protein called the von Willebrand factor, which also plays a role in clot formation. The unprocessed form of von Willebrand factor interacts easily with cell fragments called platelets, which circulate in the bloodstream and are essential for blood clotting.

By November 4, 2016, I completed the seventh TPE since my transfer to Mayo. I tolerated the procedure very well. My platelets increased slightly to 122K.

By November 7, 2016, I completed the tenth TPE since my transfer to Mayo. I experienced a mild allergic reaction to the plasma—bilateral hives on eyelids and some generalized itching on my head. They resolved it by giving me 50 mg diphenhydramine; an antihistamine mainly used to treat allergies. They completed the procedure without any further incident. My platelets increased to 141K.

On November 10, 2016, I completed my 13th TPE since my transfer to Mayo for TTP. I was premedicated with 50 mg diphenhydramine due to chronic hives on my past couple of procedures. My Platelets increased to 136K.

November 11, 2016, I completed my14th TPE since my transfer to Mayo. My Platelets were stable at 130K. At this point, the decision to do a plasma exchange was decided on a day-to-day basis. My doctor explained and I expressed the understanding of this plan.

On November 14, 2016, I completed my daily TPE. I tolerated the procedure very well. My Platelets improved to 139K, which was very encouraging.

On November 15, 2016, the consistency changed. Although I completed my daily TPE and my platelets improved to 150k, I developed a skin rash on my face, shoulder, and chest and itched uncontrollably so I was pre-medicated with Benadryl 50 mg. The nurse added Benadryl 25 mg, and my symptoms got better, but at the last unit of plasma, I developed more skin rashes with more itching. The procedure stopped, and a transfusion reaction workup ordered.

On November 16, 2016, my daily TPE was going well with pre-med of 50 mg Benadryl. The Transfusion Medicine team discussed my case during an apheresis meeting. By this time, my platelet count had risen steadily, and I reached an all high of 213K, so the doctors decided to skip a day.

On November 18, 2016, my platelet count dropped from 230 to 148 due to skipping the TPE process. Once reincorporating TPE, my platelets rose to 205k (up from 157K).

On November 21, 2016, I completed TPE, and my platelets were holding at 205k. I took a break for two days.

Thursday, November 24, 2016, would mark the first time I did not celebrate Thanksgiving with my family. Although the hospital made it possible for their patients to celebrate by serving turkey, mashed potatoes, and green beans, it just wasn't the same. However, thanks to my brother, Cavanaugh Clack, my day was made.

He brought Thanksgiving to the Mayo Clinic with his famous Cornish hens, mashed potatoes, and sweet potato pie, and to top it off, we watched football! Just what the doctor ordered! Well, it was what I needed, and I was a happy camper.

On November 25, 2016, my platelets dropped to182k. Due to persistent extremity numbness and tingling in my right lower leg, the doctors consulted neurology. I stated that since the onset of my symptoms, I experienced numbness in my right leg and tingling limited to the anterior leg.

I could not feel any sensation in my thigh or my anterior thigh, but from my patella down sensation in the right anterior leg decreased, but still had some feeling. I had some weakness more proximal in the right lower extremity; however, it improved. Since diagnosed with TTP, my weakness, and numbness improved by 25%.

On November 26, 2016, my doctor recommended that my examination was consistent with a right femoral neuropathy that was likely concerning my TTP. With physical therapy and acute rehab, they were confident that I would continue to improve. However, they would recommend an EMG if my symptoms worsened or were persistent and hadn't improved after a few weeks.

According to healthline.com, femoral neuropathy, or femoral nerve dysfunction, occurs when you can't move or feel part of your leg because of damaged nerves, specifically the femoral nerve.

When the femoral nerve is damaged, it affects your ability to walk and may cause problems with sensation in your leg and foot. This can result from an injury, prolonged pressure on the nerve, or damage from the disease. In most cases, the condition will go away without treatment.

Femoral Neuropathy

My nerve condition, femoral neuropathy has caused me difficulty in moving around. To date, my leg or knee will feel weak, and sometimes I'm unable to put pressure on my right leg. I also feel sensations as numbness on the front and inside of my thigh, tingling, and constant pain in my thigh area and around the right side of my genital region.

I have difficulty extending my knee and lifting my leg, and the craziest part is that I often feel like my leg or knee is going to give out or buckle which causes me to walk very cautiously. It's limiting my swag. Hey! I'm told that I have a very cool walk. I'm just saying.

Now even though this is still happening, I'm told that medications and physical therapy will improve my situation. However, since October 2016, when diagnosed with TTP, my symptoms have yet to dissipate.

On November 28, 2016, another TPE was scheduled and had been on a daily schedule since my platelet counts dropped significantly after holding TPE procedures on Nov 22nd and 24th. The process was followed by a dose of eculizumab (a "monoclonal antibody" that binds or attaches to a protein present in the blood used to treat aHUS).

The doctors decided to hold off on TPE for a day and resume TPE on the day after. They also decided to draw another ADAMTS13 activity and inhibitor test right before the exchange on Friday.

On November 29, 2016, my platelet count was 213. Boom! That's what I'm talking about, baby. I was so excited. At this point, it was like a game, but of course a more serious game. Each time my platelet numbers were high, I made a touchdown. Each time my platelet numbers dropped, it was like I didn't catch a pass from out of the backfield. It wasn't a good feeling.

On November 30, 2016, my platelet count was 235. However, there was a noted increase in my LDH and creatine that was particularly troubling. Earlier I stated that when your LDH rises, it means that tissues may have been damaged or are diseased.

The kidneys maintain the blood creatinine in a normal range, and as the kidneys become impaired for any reason, the creatinine level in the blood will rise due to inadequate clearance of creatinine by the kidneys. This issue could mean a possible malfunction or failure of my kidneys. The doctors decided if my labs continued to trend in the wrong direction they were going to resume TPE in the afternoon as well.

On the mornings of December 3rd and 4th 2016, I completed TPE. Soliris was tentatively planned for post TPE on the 3rd as well.

What you have read up until this point was my life at the Mayo Clinic. In addition to having treatments, getting blood drawn and numerous visits from several doctors throughout the day, my daily routine was a 4 a.m. wakeup where the nurse would take my vital signs and blood work to get my platelet count and LDH from the previous day. I would then go back to sleep.

Breakfast was at 8 a.m., and my doctors would all come in to report my numbers and discuss the game plan for the day. I would then take my morning medications. Depending on the time of my TPE treatment I would relax, read or watch TV until it was time for my wheelchair ride to transfer me to the Apheresis department.

My treatment would start with Benadryl to knock out any allergic reaction; then the plasma apheresis treatment would begin which usually lasted for about four hours. The nurse would monitor my vitals during the process, and the transfusion doctor would visit to see how I was doing and to provide a game plan or any adjustments needed based on my platelet and LDH counts.

After treatment, I would eat lunch either at the treatment site or in my room. I would recover by either sleeping or relaxing for the rest of the day.

Every couple of hours the nurse would come in to check on me, get my vitals and help with any maintenance or any care I needed. 5 p.m. would be dinnertime, and then my next scheduled medication was at 8 pm. In the meantime, I would relax.

During the day, I also had a therapist who would come in and work with me on leg exercises to help me walk better with the walker, however, the goal was to transition to walking with a cane. I worked hard while I was in the hospital. I treated it as if I were training for football and preparing for camp. After all, I was back on a structured schedule, just like my football days. Only this time I was fighting for my life.

Faith Without Works is Dead

One of the things that became most important to me was re-establishing my relationship with Christ. I started reading the Bible more; I was praying and talking to God daily, and I requested that the hospital Chaplain come and visit and pray with me as well.

My good friend and ASU teammate, turned pastor, Glen Dennard would also visit me, and we would pray. Also, another good friend and a man of God, Jon Taylor would pray with me, and of course prayers and calls from my parents and close friends were encouraging.

My relationship with God was the foundation that kept me positive and focused, and though I was going through a lot, I was grateful. I had a sense of calmness and knew that God would take care of me and guide me through my journey.

My hematology doctor, John Camoriano and I were talking, and he mentioned that as he was treating me and making several decisions and trying different treatments and medications, nothing seemed to affect me. He said to everything he wanted to try, all I would say was, "Okay let's do it." He thought to himself, "Wow! Either this guy has had so much head trauma through playing football that nothing seems to faze him or he's just out of it altogether."

Finally, he decided to ask me why I was so calm and confident about everything that I was experiencing. He said, "I'm so used to other patients being negative, always questioning things, and just giving doctors and nurses such a hard time."

I told him it was my faith in Jesus Christ. I said, "I know you are doing your job, but the final say will come from God. I trust that He will take care of me and get me through this ordeal." My doctor was like, "Wow!" That was my first opportunity to share God's goodness and my faith.

Another opportunity for me to brag about God was again with Dr. Camoriano who brought another doctor in to visit me. He shared with her the same story we discussed. He told the doctor that when I expressed my faith and trust in Jesus Christ, he made a vow to himself to do everything he could to get me healed and that my confidence in God made him reevaluate his relationship with God and the need to improve his Faith. By the time he finished telling the story, the other doctor was in tears from amazement.

Mind you, this is a high profile doctor known across the country and for me to affect him that way was such a wonderful feeling. However, most importantly that situation allowed me to share an example of how faith in God works.

James 2:14-26 states, "What good is it, dear brothers and sisters if you say you have faith but don't show it by your actions? Can that kind of faith save anyone? Suppose you see a brother or sister who has no food or clothing, and you say, "Good-bye and have a good day; stay warm and eat well"—but then you don't give that person any food or clothing. What good does that do?" Like this bible example, I showed my faith while in the hospital—professing that God had the last word—I also showed my works— staying strong, believing that God would heal me, and never wavering.

I'm Going Home! Wait.
Am I Going Home?

On December 5, 2016, my doctor came into my room and told me something that I was waiting to hear for months. He said I was being released to go home.

My platelet numbers were holding steady, and everything looked good. I was ecstatic but, on the flip side, it was a bit scary because although my numbers were up and holding, I wasn't 100% well. I still had TTP and aHUS, but they felt I was in good enough shape to be released. Not out of the dark, I still had to continue my treatments and continue as an outpatient. I was just happy to be going home.

You know the saying, "Be careful what you wish for?" Although I yearned to hear the doctors tell me I was going home, I had mixed feelings because while in the hospital nurses and doctors are checking on me 24/7 however, at home I knew I didn't have that type of care.

All sorts of questions start popping in my head. What if something goes wrong with my catheter? What if I fall down the stairs? What if no one is home and I can't drive myself to the hospital? I can't believe I'm saying this, but as nerve-wracking as it is to be stuck with needles, interrupted while sleeping, and served bland food, in my mind, the hospital was my safe place. I knew that if anything went wrong, the doctors and nurses were right there to help me.

After I went through the motions of stressing and worrying, I realized once again God's got me. Isaiah 41:10 says, " Don't be afraid, for I am with you. Don't be discouraged, for I am your God. I will strengthen you and help you. I will hold you up with my victorious right hand." That was yet another reminder that I would be okay and to not worry. So, I took heed of the scripture and quit worrying.

On December 6, 2016, one day after my release, I was re-admitted to the hospital because my platelet numbers dropped tremendously.

I stayed in the hospital for ten more days and finally released on December 16, 2016. I was free! I was on my way to recovery. I was happy that God saw fit to save me. However, I realized that Him saving me did not mean that I go back to living and doing the same things I did before my illness.

God uses sickness in our lives as a way to rebuke us, slow us down, remind us of our humanity, and to sanctify us. Also, sometimes God has us suffer physically just so that His glory is displayed in healing us. Hebrews 12:10-11 states, "…but God's discipline is always good for us so that we might share in his holiness. No discipline is enjoyable while it is happening—it's painful! However, afterward, there will be a peaceful harvest of right living for those who are trained in this way."

Out-Patient Chronicles

Buckle up because this section has more medical jargon, but worth reading.

On January 3, 2018, I returned to see my primary Dr. Nathan Delafield, as an outpatient for the very first time since being discharged from the Mayo Clinic. I felt pretty good, but honestly, no day is 100% pain-free since I retired from football. The difficulties from TTP and aHUS, the knee and back pain, and the persistent numbness to my thigh to name a few, add to my many ailments.

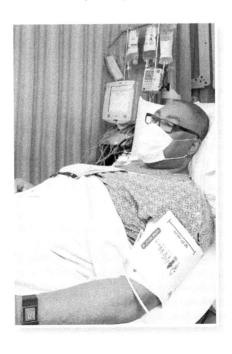

As an outpatient, my new plasma exchange (PLEX) schedule was now Monday, Wednesday, and Friday with a dose of one gram of Celcept. On Monday (after two days off of PLEX) my platelets dipped, and LDH rose, but by Friday my numbers elevated. Also, my leg was slowly getting stronger. My physical examination showed no visible skin lesions except for red patches of raised skin on my hands.

There was no physical lymphadenopathy (Enlargement of Lymph Nodes) in my cervical, supraclavicular (supraclavicular lymph node is the drainage of the mid-section of the esophagus, and lungs), axillary (the axillary lymph nodes or armpit lymph nodes drain lymph vessels from the lateral quadrants of the breast) or inguinal (inguinal lymph nodes are the lymph nodes in the groin) areas.

My ENMT (Electro Neuro Muscular Therapy) exam was ordinary. My neck was supple, without mass or thyromegaly (abnormally enlarged thyroid gland), my chest was clear to auscultation (listening with a stethoscope).

My cardiovascular examination revealed a regular rhythm without murmur, gallop (an abnormal heart rhythm marked by the occurrence of three distinct sounds in each heartbeat like the sound of a galloping horse) or rub (an audible medical sign used in the diagnosis of peri-carditis— swelling and irritation of the pericardium, the thin sac-like membrane surrounding your heart often causing chest pain occurs when the irritated layers of the pericardium rub against each other), and peripheral pulses that were full and symmetric throughout.

My neurologic exam was grossly nonfocal. A focal neurologic deficit is a problem with the nerve, spinal cord, or brain function. ... The type, location, and severity of the problem can indicate which area of the brain or nervous system is affected. In contrast, a nonfocal problem is not specific to a specific area of the brain.

My doctor noted that the aHUS/TTP overlap syndrome with doc-umented ADAMTS13 antibodies and low activity level as well as some constitutional HUS-like mutations of uncertain significance. Pointing out that on my M-W-F therapy days I did well, but my LDH and platelets were at their worst on Mondays after two days off of plasma exchange.

This report dictated that they increase my immunosuppression (Suppression of the immune system and its ability to fight infection). I was on Cellcept 1g bid so, my doctor made recommendations to increase this and alter my other medication.

On January 4, 2018, I developed a rash on my hands and wrists. Asymptomatic, but seems to be spreading up my arms. I have never had a similar rash and, I had no new exposures to food, medications, sexual partners, travel, or recent illness. There was no explanation as to why I started to develop the rash.

Dr. Ann Brewer, my dermatologist, counseled me who said it could be granuloma annular, but she was not 100% sure. This condition is idiopathic, non-life-threatening that may progress, however, it often is self-limited with one to two years.

She ordered a Biopsy for confirmation and provided me with clobetasol 0.5% cream (a topical prescription steroid used to treat the inflammation and itching caused by many skin conditions) to be used twice daily for two weeks, tapering to once daily, and then possibly every other day if tolerated until my next appointment.

To determine the cause of my condition my medications were reviewed but none seemed to be causing the granuloma annulare.

Granulomatous skin disease is in common variable immunodeficiency and HIV. My most recent HIV test was negative—something they administer periodically due to the plasma exchange I receive.

On January 9, 2018, I came in for the first of three-planned therapeutic plasma exchange (TPE) procedures. I underwent an additional exchange four days later (Saturday) because my counts had not recovered very well from the previous weekend.

My platelets were up to 230K and my LDH 302.

I had an ADAMTS13 drawn and received 50 mg IV Benadryl immediately before starting the treatment because of the several allergic reactions I'd been having from plasma.

After exchanging about two liters of the planned five liters, I developed severe itching concentrated on my hands, axilla, and back. It turns out it was Urticaria. A fancy name for a rash or hives that form on the skin as round, red blotches or welts that itch intensely caused by an allergic reaction.

The red blotches or welts can stay as small, itchy bumps or turn into large, swollen welts and can stay in the part of the body where they originated from or can spread all over the body. In my case, it was my arms and man did it itch.

Another 50 mg IV Benadryl and 10 mg liquid ranitidine (antihistamine) were added to calm down the itching. The procedure was paused for one hour while I recovered. They were able to return the extracorporeal blood without exacerbation of symptoms.

Extracorporeal blood is a procedure in which blood is taken from a patient's circulation to have a process applied to it before it is returned to the circulation. All of the apparatus carrying the blood outside the body is termed the extracorporeal circuit. Hence, Plasma Exchange—the process by which the liquid part of the blood, or plasma, is separated from the blood cells.

Typically, the plasma is replaced with another solution such as saline or albumin, or the plasma is treated and then returned to your body. After all the drama, I was discharged following a one-hour observation and was advised to notify my doctors if I noticed any more hives.

No other manifestations of allergic reactions were present (e.g., wheezing, throat swelling, cough) but because my reaction to plasma is getting more severe, the doctor's decision to try a series of 50/50 albumin /plasma (1/2protein and 1/2plasma). Jackpot! The right cocktail made the urticaria disappeared.

Come on, Man!
PTSD? Really?

" We are pressed on every side by troubles, but we are not crushed. We are perplexed, but not driven to despair. We are hunted down but never abandoned by God. We get knocked down, but we are not destroyed." – 2 Corinthians 4:8-9 NLT

After everything I had been through I was diagnosed with Post-Traumatic Stress Disorder (PTSD) to add to my list of ailments. PTSD is a condition that can occur after experiencing or witnessing a frightening, dangerous or life-threatening event, such as an unfortunate accident, war, a near-death experience, or a violent crime.

According to the American Psychiatric Association, if you are exposed to traumatic events, and then experience symptoms for more than one month, you may have PTSD.

According to the Columbia Center for Occupational & Forensic Psychiatry, some of the PTSD symptoms include re-experiencing the event; avoidance behavior; emotional numbing; inability to sleep; anxious feelings; overactive startle response; poor concentration; irritability and outbursts of anger.

Symptoms usually begin within three months of trauma, but sometimes years pass before they arise. These late symptoms are often triggered by the anniversary of the trauma or with the experience of another traumatic event.

Jessica Oifer, MA, MFT, therapy for individuals, families, and couples, says, "The symptoms of PTSD can emerge gradually over time, or they can be triggered more suddenly, perhaps by a reminder of the event. Sometimes, symptoms appear within months of the experience and other times they may take years to manifest." In my case, my symptoms appeared within a year.

Feeling agitated, moody and emotional at times, I decided to visit my doctor. His focus at this particular visit was to review my mental state because of the life-threatening event I went through and the ongoing procedures I had to go through to get better. I was having bouts of depression, and I was irritable, I had a short fuse and was taking things out on my family. I was overly aggressive with much anger.

I would isolate myself and not care about myself. I did not want to be around any friends or family. I felt sad, could not sleep, and it was difficult trying to get adjusted to being back home. Based on my doctor's examination, he diagnosed me with PTSD. — Typical for what I had been through (TTP, aHus). He suggested I see a psychiatrist.

After leaving his office, of course, I did my due diligence and researched PTSD. I read that getting timely help and support may prevent normal stress reactions from getting worse and developing into PTSD. It may mean turning to family and friends who will listen and offer comfort. It may mean seeking out a mental health professional for a brief course of therapy. Some people may also find it helpful to turn to their faith community.

Listen! At this point, I was so tired of seeing doctors that I decided to give this situation to God. Totally! I focused on prayer and letting God take care of me. I talked to Him about how I was feeling (as if he didn't know), and I asked Him to please continue to help me and heal me through this new diagnosis. My faith is strong, and I believed God heals.

If you're curious to know if you might have a touch of PTSD, an article at PsychCentral.com allows you to take a quick PTSD screening quiz to help determine if you might benefit from seeking out professional help for posttraumatic stress disorder as an adult. It takes less than a minute to complete, and you'll be provided with an instant score.

Below is the sample quiz.

Repeated, disturbing memories, thoughts, or images of a stressful experience from the past?

- o Never
- o Rarely
- o Sometimes
- o Often
- o Very Often

Feeling very upset when something reminded you of a stressful experience from the past?

- o Never
- o Rarely
- o Sometimes
- o Often
- o Very Often

Avoid activities or situations because they remind you of a stressful experience from the past?

- o Never
- o Rarely
- o Sometimes
- o Often
- o Very Often

Feeling distant or cut off from other people?

- o Never
- o Rarely
- o Sometimes

o Often

o Very Often

Feeling irritable or having angry outbursts?

o Never

o Rarely

o Sometimes

o Often

o Very Often

Having difficulty concentrating?

o Never

o Rarely

o Sometimes

o Often

o Very Often

* Psych Central warns that this is not a diagnostic quiz or professional assessment.

However, some people who take the quiz find it beneficial to talk about their symptoms with their doctor or a mental health professional (such as a psychologist). Only a properly trained physician or professional can diagnose a mental health concern.

Research shows that PTSD is often overcome; however, there are sometimes lingering effects. Living with PTSD can be an ongoing nightmare of fear, despair, anxiety and great sadness for some depending on the trauma and the individual as well as the amount of counseling but with time and treatment, most people significantly improve and are once again able to enjoy life in general.

Overtime

Most people think that being a professional football player is all glitz and glam. Unfortunately, an average player, after retiring, is likely to end up with injuries that could spiral into long-term ailments.

The key is not having a career-ending injury. However, for those players who are fortunate enough to complete their career, there are still strong possibilities that their body will sustain many types of discomforts based off of the physical abuse during our career.

Football players are at risk for injuries during and after our careers. The more I strained my body while playing, the more repercussions I'm now facing.

In my career, I've had two shoulder operations due to a separated shoulder and a labral tear. The labrum is a piece of fibrocartilage (rubbery tissue) attached to the rim of the shoulder socket that helps keep the ball of the joint in place. When this cartilage tears, it is called a labral tear.

I also had a stress fracture on my right leg where I had to wear a cast for eight weeks. Numerous cracked ribs, ankle and knee sprain on several occasions, strained back injuries, joint pain, a hip pointer (bruised hip) and of course turf toe.

When I was in the game, I focused on winning, and I was conditioned to play through pain. However, life after football is when I started to experience the effect of the injuries sustained during my career.

There have been times when I can't get out of bed.

Most mornings I roll out of bed.

However, like playing while injured, I learn to deal with this and then some. Because of these injuries, I have arthritis in both knees, both shoulders and my lower back. Wow! I'm starting to sound like an old man before my time.

I laugh about this because when I look back through the years of playing ball, there has never been a time that I've sat back and evaluated how I would feel physically after retiring. As I mentioned, I'm starting to feel like an old man, but I assume that there are many seniors today who probably feel better than me daily.

Picture this. I'm in the hospital for TTP, and I'm in the shower when my right leg buckles. I fall and can't get up. I quickly pull the emergency cord to get help.

Not thinking that a female nurse would come to my rescue—not that there's anything wrong with a female nurse seeing me naked—I had no way to cover up. Although it was a harrowing incident, it was incredibly embarrassing and uncomfortable. Something I think about when I want to laugh.

Seriously though, this is just one of those lingering physical ailments due to hits on the field that will appear unannounced. It's scary, but it keeps me on my toes.

I'm not telling you this to bash the game of football, because I love it. I'm telling you this because I want you to have a better insight into expectations during the game and long-term effects after the game.

This bit of information is also vital for women who think they want to date a professional or retired football player for the perks; parents whose children want to play football; or aspiring football players who think it's just a game when in actuality it's a life-changing experience.

No matter how well adjusted you may be, the end of a sports career is not without mental and emotional grief and physical pain.

Q & A with Marsharne Graves and Derek "DK" Kennard

n earlier chapters, I outlined my physical, emotional and mental experiences but, to give you examples of what other players go through, I administered a survey and most players had similar answers.

Former offensive lineman for Denver Broncos and Indianapolis Colts, Marsharne Graves, is experiencing ailments due to his years of playing in the NFL.

His Q & A is as follows:

Q. What injuries did you sustain while playing football?

A. My injuries ranged from concussions, broken fingers, hyperextension arms and knees, sprained ankles, fingers knees & elbows all of which came from practices and games throughout my career.

Q. Are any of those injuries affecting you currently? If so, what?

A. I suspect all the injuries I suffered from playing football has undoubtedly affected my life. For instance, my fingers, knees, and arms are continually hurting causing discomfort for the past 35 years.

Q. Do you have any physical limitations due to playing?

A. Physical limitations include no extended period of standing or strenuous lifting. Another limitation is not having the ability to drive for periods due to soreness and tightness in my knees.

Q. Physically, what has been the hardest adjustment of living everyday life?

A. Perhaps, the hardest adjustment I have to work on is keeping a positive attitude, and excepting the fact, pain and soreness are continuously are apart of my body from playing football.

Q. How often do you suffer from joint pain?

A. I suffer from joint pain daily.

Q. What do you do to alleviate the pain?

A. For me, in most situations, I try to move around and do some exercise to ease the pain by walking, stretching or riding a stationary bike.

Q. Give an example of an incident when your injury has caused a life-threatening situation?

A. My rookie year, we were playing the Atlanta Falcons in an exhibition football game during pre-season in which I was knocked unconscious and could not remember my name according to the team doctor at the time.

Q. Has your memory changed since you've retired from football?

A. Yes.

Q. What do you do to sharpen your mind?

A. I read a great deal and play board games, to sharpen my memory.

Q. Do you experience mood swings, depression, or aggression?

A. I experience aggression perhaps four to five times a week at different times of the day.

Q. Have these emotional issues affected your livelihood?

A. To some degree, my aggression has in fact over the years affected my livelihood.

Q. Would you do it again?

A. Yes, I would undoubtedly do it all over again, but this time I would play a different position such as quarterback or field goal kicker.

Another former player who agreed to take the survey is Derek "DK" Kennard, offensive linemen with Saints, Cowboys, and Cardinals. His answers are as follows:

Q. What injuries did you sustain while playing football?

A. My injuries included shoulder dislocations; shoulder separations; both elbows two surgeries each; right great toe dislocated sesamoid (a bone embedded in a tendon); right thumb was torn and dislocated; torn MCL in right knee, right knee torn patella tendon; torn right pectoral; torn left pectoral; right sciatic nerve; left sciatic nerve; neck floating debris in nerves; a slew of concussions; 90% hearing loss in right ear, ringing in the ears; seeing spots; anxiety attacks; constant pain; headaches; migraines; sleep apnea; sleep deprivation; and high blood pressure.

Q. Are any of those injuries affecting you currently? If so, what?

A. Yes all of them

Q. Do you have any physical limitations due to playing football?

A. Yes

Q. Physically, what has been the hardest adjustment of living in everyday life?

A. Living with the pain

Q. Do you suffer from joint pain?

A. Yes, daily.

Q. What do you do to alleviate the pain?

A. I use cannabis oils.

Q. What is an example of an incident where your injury could have caused a life- threatening situation. I fell asleep at a signal light!

Q. Has your memory changed since you've retired from football? If so, how?

A. Yes both long term & short term

Q. Do you experience mood swings, depression or aggression?

A. Yes, all daily and I have a short fuse!

Q. Have these emotions affected your livelihood?

A. Yes

Q. Would you do it again?

A. Not sure but, maybe if the equipment was better and we practiced as they do now, I would say yes.

I actually sent a few more guys the survey, and they agreed to participate, but they never sent the survey back. I know it's not because they were inconsiderate of my deadline, but more than likely they forgot. We tend to forget a lot, and that's one of the scariest things that many of us retired players are dealing with now in addition to our physical ailments.

Football is a love-hate sport. Even though the average NFL career lasts roughly three to five years— and the league doesn't offer guaranteed contracts—we love the game and risk it all to live out our childhood dream. Moreover, even though eligible retirees can't touch their pensions until they're 45 years old, and can't cash in their 401(k) plans until they're 59½, most of us would not change a thing.

EXOS to the Rescue

The NFL Players Association partnered with EXOS, a human performance company that helps people reach higher and achieve more. One of their services is to personalize game plans for athletes at any point in their career whether it's college, pro or retirement. Before my hospitalization, I took advantage of working out with an EXOS trainer to get my body in shape and to learn nutrition education. The program is called The Breakfast Club.

After being released from the hospital, I took it slow for quite some time. After all, I had to learn how to walk again, and to date, the femoral neuropathy is still a problem in my right thigh.

Once a year the EXOS team visits Phoenix, AZ. I looked into it and found out when they would be back in Phoenix. They offer physical therapy as well—something that I desperately needed to continue—where a board-certified physical therapist provides one-on-one care designed to treat injuries but also the overall person. Signing up for the six-week program was a no-brainer. The plan would focus on strengthening my whole body with extra work on my leg and thigh.

I worked with an excellent physical therapist, Adam Welker. No one had taken more time or effort to affect my life and increase my health and wellness like him. Before the Breakfast Club, I was unable to do some movements, but eventually, I was pushing sleds and doing kettlebell and medicine ball work. My morale even improved.

What I like about EXOS is that they tailor a program to my needs down to the food they serve after therapy or a workout. There's no "one-size-fits-all approach" as they state on their website, and they truly live up to their commitment.

To see my progress, please visit my website, **www.darrylclack.com**.

Conclusion

A llow me to reintroduce myself. My name is Darryl Clack. To date, I am coping with TTP, aHUS, first-stage dementia, depression, PTSD and femoral neuropathy. I have family and friends who love me dearly, two amazing daughters, a wife, and supportive parents.

Since my life-threatening experience, I have a renewed zest for life and a more spiritual outlook on life. Sure. I go through bouts of depression, but I take life day by day. I have a more heightened awareness of the present moment and the importance of being "in the now." I cherish every day, minute, and second I breathe, and I appreciate every hurdle that comes my way.

My story is my story. I could have kept it to myself, however, what good would that have done?

I was compelled to write this book and connect the dots to show how each illness I have relates to each other and how the common denominator is head trauma. I hope that I help as many people as possible that are suffering from the same illnesses as me or trying to find answers for their symptoms.

Countless individuals are suffering from autoimmune and rare blood diseases, dementia, PTSD, and other ailments that didn't have the chance to tell their story.

There are thousands of parents torn between letting their kids play football but have no idea where to turn for answers. Marriages are splitting up because of undiagnosed illnesses. Athletes are in turmoil because they don't know what is happening to them mentally, physically or emotionally.

I trust this book has enlightened, enriched and entertained you, and given you insight as to where to go and how to research deeper for yourself, for a friend or loved one.

I pray that after reading my story you will want to reevaluate your life and step up your spiritual game if needed. I'm not here to preach to you or put down the NFL because I love the game and I'm certainly not in the pulpit every Sunday. However, I'm here to tell my story and let you, the reader, come to your conclusion.

My life experiences—the good, the bad, and the ugly circle back to the sport that afforded me to make money, travel, enjoy the sweeter things in life and take care of my parents—Football. In football, I've been on many winning teams, but in the big scheme of things, there is only one winner. In this case, God is the winner, and I'm just a player on the team!

Many people ask me if I would do it all over again. My answer is no, and the reason is because of the pain I'm going through every day. My body aches every single day. All the surgeries I've had and all the pain medication I take is taking its toll.

I have arthritis in both knees, arthritis in both shoulders and lower back, and deal with headaches daily. I have to roll out of bed, then sit up for a few minutes and regroup my body and mind before I stand up, and these are just some of the many quirks that I live with on a regular. The game of football is hard on your body.

Some people ask me if I had a son would I let him play football. My answer is I would make sure he understood all the physical elements he would endure while playing the game and how it gets worse after the game. I would make sure he's confident and give him complete details, and if he still wants to play, then I would let him but no contact football until he gets to high school.

Do I miss the game? Honestly, I miss my teammates and the connection and closeness we had with each other. We were brothers. However, I do not miss the game such as camps and practice and all the pain and hard work my body endured. I'm good. I'm happy, and I'm alive! "Give thanks to the Lord, for he is good! His faithful love endures forever."— 1 Chronicles 16:34

Resources

Alzheimer's and Dementia Resources for Families. (n.d.). In *Approved Senior Network*. Retrieved from https://www.phoenixsenior-network.com/alzheimers-and-dementia-resources-for-families/

Big List of Alzheimer's Resources. (March 16, 2017). In *A Place for Mom*. Retrieved from https://www.aplaceformom.com/blog/list-of-alzheimers-resources-3-06-2013/

Caregiver's Guide to Understanding Dementia Behavior. (2018). In *Family Caregiver Alliance* Retrieved from https://www.care-giver.org/caregivers-guide-understanding-dementia-behaviors

Dementia Resources. (n.d.). In *American Speech-Language-Hearing Association*. Retrieved from https://www.asha.org/PRPSpecificTopic.aspx?folderid=8589935289&section=Resources

Finding Support. (n.d.). In *Memory and Aging Center*. Retrieved from https://memory.ucsf.du/finding-support

Harris, E. (2018). Top 10 Resources for Dementia Caregivers. In *Crisis Prevention*. Retrieved from https://

www.crisisprevention.com/Blog/December-2016/
Top-10-Resources-for-Dementia-Caregivers

How Connected are Concussions and Depression? In *The Globe and Mail*. Retrieved from https://www.theglobe-andmail.com/life/health-and-fitness/ask-a-health-expert/how-connected-are-concussions-and-depression/article4171563/

National Alzheimer's and Dementia Resource Center. (n.d.). In *NADRC*. Retrieved from https://nadrc.acl.gov

Online Support Group for Family Caregivers/Family. (n.d.). In American Academy of Developmental Medicine and Dentistry. Retrieved from https://aadmd.org/ntg/onlinesupportgroup

Resources Caregivers Should Know About. (n.d.). In *AARP*. Retrieved from https://www.aarp.org/caregiving/local/info-2017/important-resources-for-caregivers.html

References

Atypical Hemolytic Uremic Syndrome. (n.d.). In *National Organization for Rare Disorders*. Retrieved from https://rarediseases.org/rare-diseases/ atypical-hemolytic-uremic-syndrome/

Concussion prevention: 10 Questions to Ask Youth Sports Coaches. (October 18, 2017). In *Rise and Shine*. Retrieved from https://riseandshine.childrensnational.org/ concussion-prevention-10-questions-ask-youth-sports-coaches/

Depression in Former Professional Football Players. (n.d.). In *The Trust*, Retrieved from http://www.playerstrust.com/ mental-health/depression-former-players

D, Coldewey. (n.d.). Righteye's Portable Eye-Tracking Test Catches Concussions and Reading Problems in Five Minutes. In *Techcrunch*. Retrieved from https://techcrunch. com/2018/02/17/righteyes-portable-eye-tracking-test-catches- concussions-and-reading-problems-in-five-minutes/

D, DeNoon 1-Minute Sideline Test Predicts Concussions. (February 4, 2011). In *WebMD*. Retrieved from https://www.webmd.

com/brain/news/20110204/1-minute-concussion-test-super-bowl future#1

Femoral Neuropathy: Causes, Symptoms, and Diagnosis. (n.d.). In *Healthline*. Retrieved from https://www.healthline.com/health/femoral-nerve-dysfunction

G, Morris. (n.d.). 10 Risk Factors for Dementia. In *Activebeat. co*. Retrieved from https://www.activebeat.co/your-health/women/10-risk-factors-for-dementia/

PTSD Screening Quiz. (n.d.). In *Psych Central Staff.* Retrieved from https://psychcentral.com/quizzes/ptsd-quiz/

V, Tweed. (March 1, 2018). 10 Causes of Possibly Reversible Dementia. In *Better Nutrition*. Retrieved from https://www.betternutrition.com/features-dept/reversible-dementia

What Are the Risks of aHUS? (n.d.). In *aHUSSource*. Retrieved from https://www.ahussource.com/Patient/Risks

What Exactly is a Coma and What Happens to You When You're in One? (n.d.). In *Brain Charm*. Retrieved from https://brain-charm.com/2017/11/30/what-exactly-is-a-coma-and-what-happens-to-you-when-youre-in-one

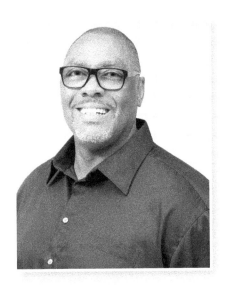

Darryl Clack Stats

- Born in San Antonio, Texas, attended Widefield High School in Colorado Springs Co.
- All-State and Prep All-America in football and track and field
- Colorado track state AAA champion in the 100,200,400 meters for three consecutive years and set state records in each that stood for 23 years before being broken
- Won three track-state titles during his career at Widefield High School
- Named Colorado Prep athlete of the year in 1982
- Inducted into the Colorado High School Hall of fame in 1993
- Inducted into Colorado Springs Hall of fame in 2006
- Attended Arizona State University from 1982-1985 on a football scholarship and ran the 100 and 200 meters on the track team
- First freshman to lead Arizona State in rushing in 30 years, in 1983
- Arizona State's 6th leading rusher in teams' history
- Won All PAC 10 honors in 1984, honorable mention ALL AMERICAN

- Named ASU football MVP
- Drafted in the 2nd round by the Dallas Cowboys in 1986 as a Running back/kick returner and played for four years 1986-1989.
- Played for Cleveland Browns during pre-season in 1990
- Played for the Canadian Football league with the Toronto Argonauts and a member of the Grey Cup championship Team 1991
- Played for the NFL World League with the Orlando Thunder
- Named team leading Rusher, and voted first team All-World honors, and the team was runner up in the World Bowl 1992
- Graduated University of Texas El Paso with a Bachelor of Science degree in Kinesiology in Sports Studies
- Graduated Organizational Management with a Masters of Arts degree from the University of Phoenix
- Has over 15 years of management experience
- Winner of 2015 Community Leadership Award sponsored by Linking Sports and Communities Cox Communications Community Volunteer Award

CPSIA information can be obtained
at www.ICGtesting.com
Printed in the USA
BVHW061927221219
567483BV00006B/14/P